IT for Health Professionals

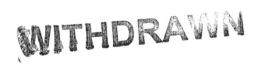

IT for Health Professionals

RUSSELL GURBUTT, MA, BSc(HONS), DPSN, PGCE, RGN

Senior Lecturer, Faculty of Health,
University of Central Lancashire

W

WHURR PUBLISHERS
LONDON AND PHILADELPHIA

© 2001 Whurr Publishers Ltd
First published 2001
by Whurr Publishers Ltd
19b Compton Terrace
London N1 2UN England and
325 Chestnut Street, Philadelphia PA 19106 USA

This text has drawn upon popular IT applications and software
as illustrations and all names used are trade marks or registered
trade marks. The programs in this book have been included for
instructional purpose on the basis of their current popularity.
They have been tested with care but are not guaranteed for any
particular purpose.

Many designations used by manufacturers and sellers to
distinguish their products are claimed as trademarks. Those
included in the text are: IBM 0S/2, Lotus Smartsuite
(International Business Machines), Internet Explorer, Windows,
Windows 3.1, Windows 98, MS DOS, Hotmail (Microsoft
Corporation), Pentium (Intel Corporation), Lycos
(www.lycos.co.uk), Ask Jeeves (Ask.co.uk), Yahoo!
(yahoo.co.uk) Netscape Navigator (Netscape), PC Plus (Future
Publishing), PC Advisor (IDG Publications), Norton anti-virus
protection (Symantec), Dr Solomons (www.drsolomons.com),
McAfee anti-virus protection (www.macafee.com), Adobe
Acrobat Reader (www.Adobe.co.uk).

British Library Cataloguing in Publication Data

A catalogue record for this book
is available from the British Library.

ISBN 1 86156 247 0

Printed and bound in the UK by Athenaeum Press Ltd,
Gateshead, Tyne & Wear.

Contents

Acknowledgements

Thanks are extended to Dawne, Jessica and Thomas Gurbutt. I would also like to acknowledge the valuable support given by Dr Martin Johnson who, as both a colleague and a manager at the University of Central Lancashire, encouraged me in a number of ways to develop both academic and research contributions in the healthcare field.

Preface

The pressure of working in the health services, along with the requirement to maintain and develop a professional knowledge base, leaves little time for staff to become seriously involved in related studies. The prospect of realistically participating in research in the workplace and collecting evidence on which to base practice is limited. Even students undertaking diploma and degree courses at a university find little time to use computer-based resources, despite their increasing availability. Moreover, if you just mention the word 'computers' to some people they 'switch off'. They find mental images of machines, 'technospeak' and having to learn a whole new way of doing things deeply unattractive.

The National Health Service aims to introduce electronic patient records, inter-professional information sharing and access to the latest guidance on clinical practice. Information technology (IT) is going to have an important impact on how professionals use information in the clinical setting. Thus there is a need to be prepared with appropriate skills to extract real benefits from using such technology. So what is the solution?

This book addresses three issues: you need basic information about how to use the computer in professional practice, you want to spend as little time as possible getting this information, and you do not want rubbish. The aims of the book, therefore, are:

- to develop your competence in using selected computer programs so that you are able to find information relevant to your professional clinical practice
- to avoid irrelevant depth of technical subject matter

- to make the best use of limited time resources whether they be at work, at home or in university-based study.

I have not included an excessive depth of technical material and have adopted the pragmatic view that to use the equipment you do not have to understand every last detail about the physics of what goes on inside it. The book will provide you with basic information about how to use the computer and troubleshoot simple problems. It will illustrate how to recognize and use applications (programs) that are useful for your professional practice, and will provide a brief guide to some selected evidence-based practice related Web sites to help you start.

Ideally you will have the use of a computer where you can sit down and practise as you work through the book. I have found that after less than 10 hours of guided study students can master basic computer skills. Soon they are surfing the Internet, sending e-mail – and discovering how to book holidays on line because the computer is a tool for both work *and* leisure, and you can apply basic computer skills to find information related to other interests such as shopping and hobbies.

I hope that you will enjoy using this book and that it empowers you to find out about current developments in your clinical field, to join in with discussions amongst peers across the world; and to use word processing skills to present your own work for publication and dissemination.

R Gurbutt
Preston
Lancashire
July 2001

Chapter 1
Choosing a computer

How to select a computer

You need to be able to judge whether the computer that you are thinking of buying will be fit for its purpose now and in the future. This will prevent you from being blinded by the salesmanship of a computer shop assistant or buying a machine that is becoming obsolete rapidly.

When buying your own computer, think about why you want to use it. If it is for simple office work, surfing the Internet and playing the occasional game then what is called an entry-level machine in the high-street store will probably give you everything that you need. Do not buy something simply because of the reassuring words of a salesperson who is earning a commission. Decide what you want and price up the best options in terms of the extras thrown in beyond your specification.

Remember that there are three levels of purchasing:

- Level one. The very latest machines with the fastest, largest capacity and the most recent features. These will cost a lot of money. They will soon become dated and, as they do so, the price will drop. These are sometimes called *power PCs* in computer magazines.
- Level two. Entry-level machines. These are capable of doing all the things that consumers currently demand, such as running an office suite of software, playing virtual games, and playing DVDs and CD ROMs. They allow Internet connection and might have a printer and scanner thrown into the package. They might be called *budget PCs* in computer magazines.

- Level three. Bargain basement or *super-budget* computers. These are machines that were yesterday's main market but are becoming obsolete. Their capacity is less than that of entry-level machines and you will need to look at what they do not offer compared with the entry-level machines. They might run older versions of software.

A second-hand computer might be sufficient to learn on, or for typing essays and reports, or producing spreadsheets and graphics but eventually it will not be adequate for the latest software and multimedia.

Some companies give away a 'free' computer if you sign up to an Internet connection package. This might seem to be attractive but the machine might not be adequate for your needs. Moreover, it is not free — you are really buying it because, with the advent of free Internet connections from companies such as Freeserve, it is now possible to obtain totally free Internet access. Some companies that provide Internet access even give free telephone access.

An example of a buyer's specification is given in Table 1.1. Once you have decided what you want then look around in computer stores and magazines to see the differences in price for the same specification. The author's experience also suggests that the after-sales service of some companies is poor. They are happy to sell you a machine but if a problem develops the telephone helpline is permanently engaged. Being able to take the computer back to a store or to talk to an engineer in the store does seem to be an important selling point. Both large and small computer shops go out of business and might not be there when you need them.

Questions to ask

- Are backup discs provided?
- Is delivery free?
- If the machine stops working is there free telephone support?
- If the machine has to be returned what are the terms?
- Does the price include someone coming round to your address to set up the computer system?

Table 1.1 A buyer's specification

Components	Spec of a machine as at 2001 (under £1200)
Desktop unit	DTU tower option
Processor (CPU)	Pentium II or Athlon 900 MHz or faster
Memory	128 MB SDRAM
Hard drive	20 GB
Zip Drive	(unlikely)
CD ROM drive	CD 40x
DVD ROM drive	16x speed (part of CD drive)
Floppy disc drive	Yes
Modem	56 K
Ports	6 USB
Monitor	17 inch, refresh rate at 1600 × 1200 resolution 75 Hz
Graphics card	32 MB memory
Sound card	Soundblaster compatible
Speakers	yes, with sub-woofers
Mouse	yes
Keyboard	yes
Software	MS Works Suite 2001, WIN DVD, Power Quest, MG1 Photo Suite, PC-cillin, Windows Me
Printer, scanner, joystick/gamepad (for entertainment)[1]	
ZIP type drives[2]	

[1] These might be included as a bundle but the higher the spec of the machine the more likely they will be purchased as extras.
[2] Purchased as an extra but the CD RW will permit 650 MB of data per CD.

The parts of a computer

If you are to choose the best computer for your needs it is helpful to know something about the parts of a computer. The computer consists of a range of different electronic components linked by cables. These are called the *hardware*. Figure 1.1 shows the typical arrangement of a desktop computer. It has a box containing the main electronic circuit boards, a monitor that looks like a small TV screen, a typewriter-style keyboard and a *mouse* – a device that

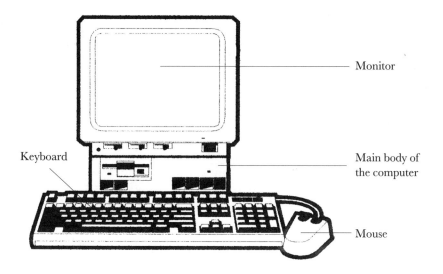

Figure 1.1 A typical desktop personal computer.

controls an electronic pointer on the monitor screen. These will now be discussed in greater detail.

Monitor

This looks like a television screen but in fact is far superior to it in terms of the picture it produces. The trend is towards flat-screen monitors rather than bulky cathode ray tubes. Flat screen monitors occupy less space on your desk (called the *footprint*) and are better for the eyes of the user. At the time of writing they are expensive but eventually their price will fall.

The monitor can display different colours as a result of a component inside the computer called the *video card*. The capacity of the video card is measured in megabytes (MB). To play games and use audio-visual media such as film clips you will need sufficient memory on the video card. The typical capacity of a computer video card to handle images is 8 MB.

The desktop unit

The main body of the computer is housed in a box that contains all the electronic circuits and pieces of wizardry that translate your commands into actions. This box is either horizontal or stands upright – in the latter case it is called a *tower*. If you are really curious about what is contained in it then have a look in the resources section for a fuller explanation and links to other sources of technical information. Remember that it is not essential to know what goes on inside the computer but it is necessary to know how to operate it.

The capacity of the computer is expressed in terms of *speed* and *memory*. To be able to adapt to do new types of work in the future it might be necessary to increase this capacity. This is commonly called being *upgradeable*. Computers can be upgraded in terms of their memory, speed, their monitors, their video and graphics cards, sound cards and so forth. However, the falling prices of computers and the rapid development of their capabilities mean that it might actually be as cheap to buy a new computer as to upgrade an old one.

Processor speed

The computer's main component is the central processing unit (CPU). This is a microprocessor chip. Its speed is expressed in hertz (Hz). Many chips are made by two companies, Intel and AMD. They are often marketed under a brand name such as Intel Pentium III 600. In the early 1990s a 33 MHz or 66 MHz speed CPU was the norm. At the end of the 1990s, 600 MHz to 1000 MHz (called a gigahertz (GHz)) speeds were common. Generally speaking, the faster the speed of the processor the faster the computer will work for you, although the other components also have an effect on the overall speed of operation.

Memory

The memory is akin to a temporary store where work is sent to be done while the CPU is busy with other activities. The larger the memory size the more able it is to free up the CPU to do other tasks. Memory is expressed in MB. If you want to play games then you will often need 64 MB of memory or more. The RAM memory is only a temporary store and is erased when the computer is switched off.

The permanent memory for storage is the hard drive. It is usually called the 'C' drive on a personal computer and its storage capacity is also expressed in terms of MB or gigabyte GB. It is a fixed component that contains all the programs loaded on to the computer and any work that you save. An IBM personal computer from the early 1990s had a capacity of just 40 MB. A PC hard drive in the year 2001 could be as large as 30.7 GB and a typical mid-range machine might have a 14.2 GB hard drive.

The CPU and memory chips fit into the main circuit board, called a *motherboard*. It also has other slots for fitting more cards (small circuit boards with memory and processing chips). These can include a sound card, a graphics card and a modem (see below). The sound card enables you to hear audio material, the graphics card enables you to play visual media and the modem allows the computer to communicate with other computers.

The modem

A *modem* passes information from your computer along a telephone line and is converted by another modem at the destination computer so that the information can be read. Faster modems have been developed over time. Their speed is expressed in kilobits per second (Kbps). Faster modem speed will mean that you are spending less time using the telephone line to send the information and means that the costs of telephone use will be lower over time.

The modem is classified according to the speed at which it transfers data to and from the network. Information is transferred in the form of bits. Eight bits equal one byte. The speed of information transfer is expressed in *bits per second*. The more bits that are transferred per second the greater the speed of the modem.

Another term that is used to describe the speed of a modem is *baud rate*. This is a measure of how many changes in tone (or frequency) can occur in one second. The average computer user is not concerned with the subtle differences in these definitions and the two words are often used interchangeably. Some common modem speeds are 56 Kbps and 90 Kbps.

The popular term for using a telephone line from your computer is *being online*. When you disconnect from the telephone it is called *being offline*. There has been a move to allow free telephone usage for computer users on the Internet in the UK but this will develop only if it is a viable business option. Until that time there are deals on offer such as one penny per minute online charges.

Removable disc drives

If you look at the front of the desktop unit there are a number of slots where you can insert discs such as a 3.5-inch floppy disc, a CD ROM or a DVD ROM. These are called drives, the floppy disc drive usually being called the 'A' drive and the CD ROM drive being called the 'D' drive. You might have a larger-capacity drive such as a ZIP drive, which has removable discs of 100 MB or 250 MB capacity. The handling of discs and storage of data is covered in Chapter 4.

The keyboard

The keyboard is the means by which you give the computer commands to perform actions. You can also buy touch-sensitive screens where you press on a particular point and the screen image changes, or you can, with some programs, talk to the computer and get it to type whatever you say. Many keyboards are connected to the back of the computer with a lead. Some use infra-red beams instead of a lead. These work in the same way that a TV remote control handset works.

The mouse

Another means of giving commands to the computer is to use a mouse. This is basically a ball in a plastic housing that has a couple of command buttons. It is either connected to the computer with a wire or uses an infra-red beam. The mouse, when slid over a mouse mat, moves an electronic pointer across the monitor screen (the mouse should be used with a mouse mat so that the moving ball has a surface to onto to ensure that it rotates). The buttons, when pressed, will either initiate an action or display a menu containing a list of choices of actions that you can take. These buttons can perform the same actions as the 'return' or 'enter' keys on the keyboard.

If you find moving a mouse about a mouse mat too uncomfortable on your wrist then there are static mice, which have the ball on top and you use a finger tip to rotate the ball to move the pointer across the screen. Personally I find these easier to use. Other options include a special pen and tablet: moving the pen point across the tablet moves the mouse pointer across the monitor screen.

Printer

There are several other peripheral devices that can be connected to the computer, such as scanners, video recorders, digital cameras and printers. The printer will be discussed as this is the most common piece of peripheral equipment that you will use.

There are two main types of printer: the ink-jet and the more expensive laser printer. Ink-jet printers are the printers of choice for home use. Laser printers are faster, often provide better quality printing, and are suited for organizations.

Ink-jet printers are quite inexpensive, some being as cheap as £50. They can be black and white or colour and they can print photo-quality images. The points to look for are the ability to handle different paper sizes such as envelopes, banners and cards as well as A4 sheets. Image reproduction is expressed in dots per inch (dpi) and speed is expressed in pages per minute (ppm). It can be tedious waiting for a 50-page report to print out at 2 ppm. The ink cartridges are also quite expensive and when deciding on a printer it might be worth considering one that has refillable cartridges and so will be more economical in the long term. Colour cartridges mix three separate chambers of ink and it might be better to choose one where you can fill individual chambers. It is worth considering this if you are paying £15–£25 per cartridge. A refill sachet could be as little as a third of this price.

Connections between the hardware components

Cables are the most obvious connections cluttering up the work desk. They include cables for power, the monitor, the mouse, the keyboard, the printer, the speaker and the modem. You might also have a microphone and a game pad or joystick that also require cables. These will all plug into sockets, called *ports*, at the back of the computer.

There are different types of ports: parallel, serial, USB, speaker and modem cable ports. It is important to know where each lead fits. Your computer's instruction manual will tell you this but it is not hard to work it out because the different cables will plug into only certain ports. Some desktop units have symbols or words next to the ports to guide you as to which lead fits where.

Software

So far we have looked at the *hardware* or the physical components of the computer. This section looks at the *software* – the programs that make the physical components do work. Software is the name given to programs written in a language that the processor understands and to which it can respond. You do not need to know the programming language – just how to use a keyboard and mouse.

The first software program to know about is the operating system for the computer. Common ones are IBM OS2, MS DOS, Windows 3.1, Windows 95, Windows 98, and Windows NT. The operating system does just what it says – it allows the computer to work and determines how you are able to give it commands. The meeting place between operating system and the computer user is at the graphical user interface (GUI). This is the screen image that you see when you input a command instruction. You might do this by placing the mouse pointer over a small picture called an *icon* and clicking the mouse button to make the computer start a given program. Good GUIs make computers very easy to use – ideally you should be able to work out what to do just by looking at the screen. Formerly an operator would have to learn a list of command words to type in. That is now mostly a thing of the past and the sort of commands demonstrated in this book will be simple point-and-click commands using a mouse to make the computer do something. You will find that it is as easy as operating a TV remote-control handset. If you have your own PC then you should have a copy of the operating system software on a CD ROM. This allows you to reload it if something damages the current system configuration.

Application software

The operating system is the main software that allows you to use any other programs that you load on to the computer. These other programs are called *applications* and they include programs such as an office or drawing application, games, Internet browsers and e-mail programs.

Drivers

A third type of software is a *driver*. This is a small program that allows the computer to recognize and operate a particular piece of hardware. Drivers will often be supplied on 3.5-inch floppy discs with the hardware, be it a mouse, printer or CD ROM drive. Some operating systems will automatically recognize newly installed hardware without you having to take any action. Others will display an on-screen message asking you to insert the driver disc and load the program on to the hard drive.

Multimedia software

There is a kid in all of us and the computer can be used for entertainment: computer games can let you race a car at Le Mans or join in a Star Wars galactic battle. Most games include sound as well to add to the realism. Games can be useful for just gaining confidence in using a limited range of basic functions of the computer, but in professional terms the *edutainment* resources you can buy are probably of more value. Edutainment means education that is enjoyable. It includes commercial CD ROM of encyclopaedias, atlases, and clinical resources produced by major journal publishers and academic institutions. For example you could buy a CD containing archives of several years of full-text copies of a clinical journal.

Computers for communication

Computers can communicate with each other; but they can have problems receiving and processing information.

Physical barriers to communication include hardware damage, loose cables and interruptions to the telephone line connections. Sometimes the dialup connection is too busy to permit you to be connected, for example. Other barriers involve the impairment of the operating system and other software. This is most commonly caused by virus attacks or software incompatibilities so that systems cannot communicate information even if physically connected to a network.

Networks

A single computer is called a *stand-alone unit* but if it is physically connected to one or more other computers it is called a *networked computer*. A simple network has several terminals that people use to connect to one 'main' computer, which is called a *server*. The terminals are *clients*.

Hospitals and universities will commonly have networks of computers. An example of a hospital network is a computer-based outpatient appointment record system. Networks that allow users to communicate with other users on the network are called *intranets*. If the network was connected to the world outside of the hospital or the university then it would be called an *extranet*. A desktop PC can be connected to other computers across the world via a telephone connection. This is called the *Internet*.

The future of information technology

At the time of writing, the latest computer developments for entertainment involve digital television, which allows Internet access with minimal skill requirements through the television using a portable keyboard or a handset. The commercial impetus for this is electronic shopping (*e-tailing*). However, for professional use you will also need some means of storing information, writing your own documents and communicating with other professionals.

If you want to keep abreast of what is happening in the computer market then there are a range of magazines available at newsagents, some of which include CD ROMS containing software attached to them. Some focus on entertainment whilst others are more technologically oriented. *Which Computer* is a good guide for buying and evaluates products. *PC Advisor* usually has a range of (free) popular leisure software such as encyclopaedias. *PCPLUS* is for the serious computer buff and the free CD ROMs contain useful tutorials and software. The greater part of most computer magazines consists of advertising material but the free software alone is sometimes a good enough reason to buy.

Chapter 2
Setting up a computer system

Introduction

Chapter 1 introduced you to the essential components of a computer system. This brief chapter leads you through the process of setting it up so that it works. Chapter 3 explores what you see on the screen once the computer has completed its start-up sequence.

If you have your own PC it should have a manual that leads you through a few simple steps to ensure that it is set up correctly. If you are buying a PC and someone comes to set it up for you, ensure that you have some detailed information about how to do this. You might want to move the computer to another room or another house – this will entail removing leads and refitting them.

There are three main things that will stop your computer from working correctly. The first is that the simple connections are not securely in place. That is easily remedied. The second is that the hardware components have a fault, in which case you will need technical advice. Third, the software might be corrupted, for example by a virus. This can be dealt with using anti-virus programs and by reloading software applications.

As with any machine, things can and do go wrong. Look at the simple things first before resorting to technical help. It is important for you to develop the confidence to undertake simple fault tracing and to know when to seek external advice from a colleague, workplace technician or telephone support helpline.

First check that you have fitted the cables and leads correctly. Setting up a computer system is relatively straightforward. All you really need to remember is to ensure that the correct leads are properly inserted into the correct sockets. With a typical desktop PC you will need to ensure that the following cables are in place:

- a power lead from a socket connected into the desktop unit;
- a power-supply lead from a socket into the back of the monitor;
- a connecting lead from the desktop unit to the back of the monitor;
- a lead connecting the mouse to the desktop unit;
- a lead connecting the keyboard to the desktop unit;
- a cable connecting the printer to the desktop unit;
- a lead and possibly power supply to external speakers;
- a telephone lead from a telephone socket to the modem port in the desktop unit (if fitted).

You will notice that plugs at the ends of different leads are designed in different ways. Some have a three-lead ending, others a series of pins. Basically, you can't fit the wrong terminal into the wrong socket – it's that easy. You could make a note, or draw a diagram showing where each lead should fit on your computer for future reference.

There are different types of socket that fit into different ports. These are: serial ports, parallel ports, USB ports and the power-supply socket.

Mice and keyboards can have either PS2 or USB connections and it is important that you buy peripherals that are compatible with the sockets in your desktop unit. You can buy adapters to permit the connection between, say, a PS2 mouse and a desktop unit port.

Some connection leads have small screws that firmly anchor the lead into the socket. It is important to screw these equally otherwise you might distort the pins on the lead of the base unit. More recent designs have a peg that you turn to tighten the screw, others require a fine-bladed screwdriver. Printer leads tend to have wire clips that hold the connection on to the printer.

Having made sure that these are firmly connected you are then ready to switch the power on at the socket (if it has a switch), the 'power on' button on the desktop unit and the 'power on' button on the monitor. The next thing that should happen is that the computer commences its own checks and runs through a sequence of actions that eventually load up a screen, which is called your 'desktop'. This process is called 'booting up'.

Troubleshooting to diagnose why the system is not working

Assuming that you have connected up the cables, or they are already connected, and that you switch the computer on – the following might happen:

- *Nothing happens when the base unit switch is pressed to boot up the computer.*
  - Check that the mains power is switched on.
  - Check that the mains power cable is firmly pushed into the base unit socket. Press the 'on' switch again on the base unit and check to see if the small light on the front of the unit glows indicating that the system is booting up. You will probably hear whirring noises as disc drives operate and the system performs a series of checks.
- *The base unit is operating but there is nothing on the monitor.*
  - Check that the monitor is switched on.
  - Check that the monitor mains power is switched on.
  - Check that the monitor cables are firmly pressed into their respective sockets. These cables will consist of a power supply cable and a cable joining the monitor to the base unit.
- *The boot up screen information appears but then stops.* Check that you have not left a disc in the 3.5-inch floppy disc drive. If you have, remove it and press the 'return key'. (The system will have been trying to boot up from the floppy disc.) The boot up procedure should then continue.

If these simple steps do not resolve your problems then either consult the manuals that were delivered with the computer, which will contain a troubleshooting section, or if it is a workplace machine, consult the technical support staff. Helpdesk telephone advice is often available within large organizations, and user and technical support should be part of the package if you have brought a new computer.

You might want to check that the computer is set up and boot it up ready for the introduction to the desktop and applications covered in Chapter 3.

Chapter 3
The healthy computer

Introduction

This chapter will discuss the computer in normal use. Some of the functions that will be examined have been selected because of their relevance to seeking, collating and recording the information that you might use in professional practice. The Windows 98 operating system will be used as the example of a typical desktop screen and the principles of its operation will be discussed. If you want full details on this operating system then there are a number of books

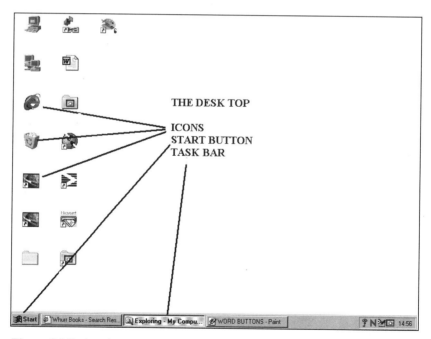

THE DESK TOP

ICONS
START BUTTON
TASK BAR

Figure 3.1 Desktop image.

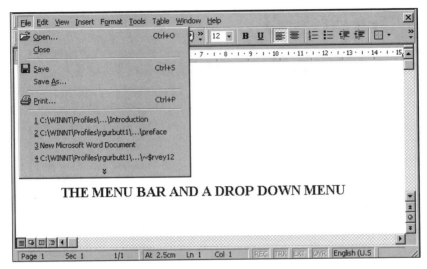

Figure 3.2 Drop down menu image.

that describe its features. You can also try the help files in the menu bar or there might be an introductory tutorial in the program files.

The keyboard

The keyboard has a 'qwerty' format typing section, a 0–9 number pad and a series of function keys – F1 to F12. The function buttons are short cuts to activities such as save, spell check and help topics. There are three *hot keys* that, when depressed together, will restart the computer. These are the 'ctrl', 'alt' and 'delete' keys. If your computer suddenly stops working (called *crashing* or *hanging up*) there are a couple of strategies that can be employed, which will be discussed below. The important thing is not to switch the power supply off and on again. This will lose any work that you have not saved, and can affect the software operation. Having said that, modern operating systems do have some functions that recover the system after a crash. The other main keys to be aware of are the 'return' and 'enter' keys. These have the same function as a left click of the mouse.

The mouse

The mouse has two, and occasionally three, buttons and sometimes a wheel for scrolling the pointer up and down the screen. There are several functions that you can perform with a mouse. These are: point, left and right click, select, drag and drop.

Pointing

If you move the mouse then you will see the pointer on the monitor screen move in a corresponding manner. The pointer is usually an arrow but some software can allow you to change it to other objects. You might notice that sometimes the pointer changes into a flashing vertical bar (called the cursor) and at the side of a window it changes to a double-ended arrow. The use of these functions will be discussed under the 'windows' section.

The terms *click, left click* or *single click* mean to press and release the left mouse button once. A *double click* means to press and release the left mouse button twice in rapid succession. *Right click* means to press and release the right mouse button. The two buttons left click and right click give the computer an instruction to undertake a given activity. (Note that if you are left handed then you can set up the mouse to reverse the buttons, this book however assumes that the mouse is set up for right handed users.) If you 'right click' when the pointer is over an object then a menu will appear offering a range of possible actions. These will be covered in more detail later in this chapter. Left clicking when the pointer is over an object will launch that application – again this is discussed later in this chapter.

Drag and drop

Drag and drop is used to copy or move an item across the screen or across applications. You select text by holding down the left mouse button and dragging the pointer over it. The text is now selected and will be shown as a black shaded area. To move it to the right, click over the shaded area and, whilst keeping the button depressed, drag the portion of text to your required location. Releasing the mouse button will drop it in that place. This will be demonstrated in the section about using the word processor.

To move an object, such as an icon, right click over it and whilst keeping the button depressed drag the object to another location. Then release the button to drop the object in its new place. Right clicking over an object will reveal a pop-up menu with a range of options such as 'open', 'explore', 'send to', 'cut', 'copy', 'create shortcut', 'delete', 'rename' and 'properties'. You can also move it using the menu commands.

Selected applications

There are three key applications that will help in developing your knowledge and resources to support evidence-based practice. These are:

- word processing;
- Internet browsing (searching);
- e-mail.

Word processing skills will enable you to keep records and write reports about your clinical resources and research. Information to develop insight into your area of research or clinical interest, for example, can be accessed through using an Internet browser. Once you have access to a number of sources such as journals and professional organizations you can then use the e-mail facility to communicate with other professionals, journal editors and discussion groups to share information and find out about conferences and other events relevant to your area of interest. Of course, apart from professional uses, the Internet provides a wealth of useful information, from holidays, finance and shopping to railway timetables. Over the next few years, as the technology becomes easier to use and cheaper to obtain, the number of people using electronic media as part of their working and leisure time is set to rise. Knowing how to use the technology effectively will allow you to maximize the benefits it has to offer relating to your personal and professional development.

Word processing

What is it?

A word processor is an application that allows you to create and alter a document easily. Examples of word processing applications are Microsoft Word for Windows, Lotus Word Pro and Claris Works.

What does it do?

Word processing allows you to create a document, type words (text) and then to be able to alter them in various ways, including making changes to the type face, the size and the spacing, or to make it appear bold or underlined or in italics. All the things that were formerly done using a typewriter can be achieved using a word processor but there are far more advantages to the latter.

The document you create can use a predesigned template such as a business letterhead or memo that you select and use. Tables and pictures can also be added into the page, as can page numbers and a whole range of options for paragraph spacing and alignment. You can even check whether your spelling and grammar are correct.

Some advanced applications such as 'voice type' even allow you to talk to your computer, which then types out your dictation. However, for the purposes of this book we shall concentrate on being able to master manual word processing. When you come to printing out your work you have a number of options. You can press a button that will instruct your printer to print off a copy. This is called a *hard copy*. Alternatively you can send it as an attachment to an e-mail letter, which transmits your document with a covering letter to someone else's computer. They can then read it and print their own copy, or type in alterations and e-mail it back to you. Finally, you can store your work on a floppy disc or a CD ROM and take it to another computer to continue the work at a later date. Electronic storage means that there should be less need for reams of paper, and it makes your work more portable.

What is it used for in professional practice?

If research evidence is to be used as a means of underpinning aspects of your practice then a word-processed document can be a good resource to disseminate information and analyses of papers reviewed, produce reports or type articles for publication.

If you are undertaking primary research or an academic course then word processing will be an invaluable means of writing up your report, essay, dissertation or thesis.

If you are building a resource base of evidence and practice related to your area then a word-processed portfolio can be used to detail the resources and contacts drawn upon as well as being able to be updated periodically. This can also be shared among interested groups using e-mail.

Finally, the requirement to maintain professional portfolios and to update your knowledge base periodically can be documented in word-processed files, which can be augmented and printed out as required.

Internet browser

What is it?

The browser allows you to look at resources on the Internet. Examples are Microsoft Internet Explorer and Netscape Navigator.

What does it do?

The browser allows you to navigate from page to page in documents on the Internet. The documents can be anywhere in the world and you can move from one to the other by the click of a button. This can be likened to visiting a library in London where you go and select a book from a particular shelf, open it at a given page and read a specific passage. However in reading that page you see a word that opens up another line of enquiry. You can then with the click of a button visit another library in New York and select a book on a set shelf and view a set page. That, in turn, leads you down another line of enquiry and allows you to view the page of a book in Hong Kong. Without the Internet it would be possible to obtain copies of these books on inter-library loan but by using the Internet you can browse right across the world at the click of a button. Anything that you find interesting can be printed or stored electronically on your computer.

What use is it for professional practice?

The problem with evidence for practice is to know what evidence is available and to know how other professionals are conducting their practice. Attending conferences and presentations and making visits are some ways of finding out, but they incur costs and take time that might not be available. The Internet can play a role in providing access to collections of journals called *databases,* which you can search for material related to your topic. For example, you could be working with oncology patients and want to know about current developments in a particular field of oncology regarding the advice currently being issued. With a few clicks of a button, and after typing in some search words relevant to your enquiry, you will produce a list of pages and databases to view. You then choose to browse whichever is most relevant.

In the UK there are a number of medical databases and electronic libraries and journals 'online' that give you access to material directly related to healthcare practice. There are also the political (Department of Health, Department of Social Security) and professional Web sites (BMA, UKCC), which allow you to read full text documents and commentary on current health-related issues.

You can access these resources either at work or at a home on a PC connected to the Internet.

Once you are in possession of information you then are in a stronger position to undertake your own critical review and evaluation of relevance to your practice. Remember, it is still important to read critically anything you obtain from the Internet, as you would with a professional journal. It provides you with information but it does not do the thinking for you.

E-mail

What is it?

It is electronic mail, a means of sending messages to another computer user electronically. Recipients receive e-mails in their mailbox on their computer or e-mail-enabled machine such as a mobile telephone. Electronic mail allows you to send messages, add priority symbols, attach documents and pictures and join in discussion groups involving a number of people.

What use is it for professional practice?

It permits rapid communication with other professionals whom you might otherwise not meet. This can be good for networking. You can exchange documents, seek peer reviews, send electronic conference abstract submissions and set up automatic mailing services that update you about the latest contents of current journals. If you are requesting information on a topic it can be sent as an attachment to an e-mail message. That attachment can be opened and read in a word processing application.

Windows

Navigating around the desktop and taskbar

Boot up your computer and use the mouse and keyboard to navigate your way around the desktop screen. The first activity is to look at what you have on the desktop. There is a task bar along the base of the screen and a start button in the left-hand corner. A series of *icons* (small pictures) are visible on the screen above the task bar and these are the recycle bin, the Internet application, the mail application and a 'my computer' application.

How to shut down the computer

A menu will appear if you left click on the start button. The most important selection is the 'shut down' button. You need to shut your system down correctly so that you do not lose your work or damage the software programs. To shut down the computer you click on this selection and a menu (or dialogue box) appears with some options. You can choose only one. The round button with a dot is called a *radio button*. Click on the button that you want to select. Then click OK to confirm your action for what you want the computer to do. Pressing 'ctrl' plus 'alt' and 'delete' will also restart the computer. You can always click on 'cancel' in the dialogue box if you select shut down by mistake. Once the computer has shut down it will either automatically switch off the power or display a message saying that it is safe to turn it off.

Finding files, folders and programs on your computer and removable discs

There are several ways in which this can be done and these are discussed next. To find programs click on the 'start' button and then on 'programs'. This will reveal a list of the programs installed on your computer. Move the pointer across these to select the one that you required. Notice that the selected program will be shaded in blue when the mouse pointer is placed over it. To launch the program just click on it. Click on the word-processing application by locating it from programs in the start menu.

Using Windows Explorer

Windows Explorer is a file management program that is located in the programs files found via 'start'/'program'/'Windows Explorer'. When opened it displays a window with two panes. The left-hand pane lists all the folders under each drive and the desktop. Clicking on one of the drive letters will expand its contents and display all the contained folders and files. The right-hand pane will display the contents of whatever drive or folder is selected in the left-hand pane. To select a drive or folder just click on it once. It will show the folder title in a blue shaded bar indicating that it has been selected. To open a file just click on the one required in the right hand pane. The application containing that file will launch and display the file.

Using the 'find files or folders' program

If you know the file that you want but cannot remember exactly where it is stored then there is a 'find files or folders' program in 'start'/'find files or folders'. When you launch this, a small dialogue box with a search facility will appear. You type in the name of the file required in the indicated field, select the drive on which you want to search for it and then click on 'find now'. If you are unsure which drive to select then the 'browse' button will reveal a list of your options. Select one and the 'look in' field will display your selection. Once you click on 'find now' the search will commence and all files of that name will be recorded in a window that appears at the base of the dialogue box. Leaving the 'named' field blank will display all of the files on a selected drive.

The recycle bin

You will see an item called the recycle bin. If you have a file that you no longer need then you can drag and drop it on to your recycle bin. Clicking on the bin will open a window showing its contents and then you can select 'empty recycle bin'. This will delete the contents. Do not delete unwanted programs in this way – use an uninstall utility.

You can send a file to the recycle bin by right clicking on it on the desktop and selecting the delete command from the pop-up menu.

Shortcuts

A shortcut is an icon that can be created and placed wherever you require to provide easy access to launch a frequently used application. An example might be the Word icon, which is stored away in the programs folder. A small menu will appear when you release the right mouse button. Select 'create shortcuts here' and the icon will appear on the desktop. To put a shortcut copy of this icon on the desktop all you have to do is click on 'start'/'programs' and hold the mouse pointer over 'Microsoft Word'. Right click on 'Microsoft Word' and a menu will pop up. Select 'move here' and a copy of the icon will appear. Next right click and drag the icon and release it over a space on the desktop.

You can right click over an icon and drag it to the task bar and select 'move here' when you release the mouse button. The icon will then be available on the task bar.

Familiarizing yourself with a window

A window is a rectangle that is a popular means of displaying the interface of a program. Windows have a similar layout, which includes the following.

Title bar

The top bar of the window is called the title bar. It is usually coloured blue but this can be altered according to your preferences. The title bar shows the name of the program and the file currently being worked on.

Resizing and controlling the size of the window

The title bar has three buttons in the top right hand corner – a dash, a rectangle and a cross. The function of the dash is to 'minimize' the window. When you click on this it will not close the window but rather reduces its size or stores it away on the taskbar until you next require it. To restore it to the original window size then just click on the taskbar button. If you right click over a minimized application on the taskbar button then a menu will appear that gives options such as 'restore', 'maximize' or 'close'.

The rectangle on the title bar when clicked will enlarge the window to fill the whole screen. In this case the rectangle changes into two overlapping rectangles. Clicking on this again returns the window to its previous size.

The cross button closes the window. If this is an application where you need to save work then a reminder box will appear giving you the opportunity to do this.

The size of the window can be altered easily. To do this you move the pointer over the edge of the window until it changes into a double-ended arrow. Hold the left mouse button down to select the margin of the window and drag it to the size required. You might have a shaded portion in the right hand corner of the window. If you click and drag this, the window can also be increased or decreased in size.

Menu bar

This is a list of menu headings that open up drop-down menus when clicked. A program can be closed in two ways. Click on 'file' and 'close' in the menu bar, or the cross control button on the title bar, or by right clicking on the title bar and selecting close. In each case you will be prompted to save your work.

Tool bars

These are buttons that provide quick access to menu items at a single click. Applications will have a series of pre-set toolbars that can be displayed or hidden. These are controlled through the 'view' menu and clicking on 'toolbars'. All you do is click on the check boxes for the ones you require. Click OK and they appear in your window. Right clicking on the toolbar area will also launch this menu to alter your selection.

The bar at the base of the window provides information about the contents of the window and might have some icons or additional menu words.

Switching between programs

If you have more than one application open at once they will be laid over each other on your desktop rather like sheets of paper placed over each other on a physical desk. You will know what is open by looking at what is displayed on the taskbar. To switch between programs you just click on the one that you require. Another way of switching between programs is to use the keyboard and hold down 'alt' and then press 'tab'. This will display the programs you have open. Pressing the 'tab' button will alter the highlight box from one icon to the next. Releasing 'alt' will switch you to the highlighted program.

Scroll bars

Scroll bars will usually be visible on the side and base of the window. These appear in some windows when there is more information than is visible on the screen. To view material 'off' the screen click on the scroll arrows to move up or down. The double scroll arrows take you to the top or bottom of the screen document. The 'page up' and 'page down' keys will perform the same function. If you click the mouse pointer on the screen and use the 'up' and 'down' arrows on the keyboard the screen will scroll line by line. You can also click and drag the small square on the scroll bar to control this function.

If you have several windows open you will notice that the window that is currently being used (the *active window*) has a blue title bar. The other inactive windows have a pale grey title bar. If you switch windows to work in one of the others, when you click on it the title bar will show as blue (indicating that it is the active window) and the one that you have left will show a grey title bar. You can move the active window by dragging the title bar and releasing the window wherever you want it. If you close the word-processing application by clicking 'file', 'exit' you will return to the desktop screen.

Some other resources

Setting up the mouse for left-handed use

Click on 'start', 'settings', 'control panel' and then on the mouse icon in the window which opens. This will open a mouse 'properties' window, which allows you to alter the settings and speed at which the mouse responds to clicks.

Where do I find out what the function keys do?

Look in the 'help' menu, click on the 'answer wizard' and type in 'shortcut keys'. Click on search and select the 'shortcut keys' line. A list will appear and from that select 'function key shortcuts'. This will lead you to a detailed listing of what each key will do.

Chapter 4
Word processing

Introduction

When preparing memos, reports, or documents for publication, the huge advantage of a PC is that you have a great deal of flexibility in drafting and revising your work. It can be sent electronically to a tutor or colleague for comments, or as a memo prior to meetings. You can even send articles for journal publication via e-mail and know that they have arrived. You do not have to be a typist in order to word process a document. One- or two-finger typing is often sufficient. Who really cares if real typists snigger so long as you achieve the result you want? Indeed, with practice you can achieve quite a reasonable typing speed and then you can spell-check afterwards. For those who are real technophiles then 'voice type' software allows you to talk to your computer and it types out what you say. Some market commentators see this as the way ahead in computer development. The days of the keyboard and touch screen may be limited. This section, however, will focus on keyboard-based word processing.

The days of handwritten or even typewritten submissions are passing and the norm is to produce your work using a word processor. If this is new to you this chapter will provide you with an introduction that will enable you to produce well-presented text documents. If you are familiar with using a word processor then you might want to browse through this section and use it as a refresher or to pick up hints and tips.

Even if you feel that this chapter is familiar material please read the section about file management. It is a necessary part of any IT work and it is essential that you maintain good practice so that you do not lose files that represent many hours of work. Unfortunately, at some time you will experience a computer crash or the effect of a computer virus and be concerned as to where all your hard work has gone. A few minutes' reading could save you a great deal of time.

Desktop publishing

The advent of computers radically changed the publishing industry. There was a time when teams of typesetters used metal characters to construct pages of a publication and these were mechanically imprinted on to metal plates, which were used with inked rollers, over which the paper passed. It was a long process and involved several people. Now you can be the author, editor, typist and print manager just by sitting at your own desktop, laptop or palmtop.

Introduction to disc drives

Your PC will have a number of places where information can be stored permanently. These are called the *drives*. On a stand-alone PC you will have the main internal drive, called the *hard drive*, and that is usually assigned the letter 'C'. There will often be a removable disc drive which uses 3.5-inch 1.44 MB floppy discs and that is usually called the 'A' drive. If you have a CD ROM bay on your PC, that is often called the 'D' drive. The reason I say 'often' is that the letters can be changed. If you plug in a zip drive you can add the capability of working with a 100 MB or 250 MB discs. That would probably be the 'E' drive. Computer users working on a network such as in a hospital or a university will be assigned a server space designated by a letter, for example 'F'. The importance of all this is that when you are producing documents it is necessary to know where your work is stored, not only from the practical point of view of finding it again but also from a privacy perspective. Having said that, you can always set up password protection to bar access to your files.

Current developments include facilities to store information on CD ROMs that contain about 600 MB of data. However, for the purposes of the PC user without a CD rewriter we shall confine ourselves to the most common means of storing data: the 'C' and 'A' drives.

Handling discs

If you are using floppy discs then it is important to handle them correctly, not to touch the magnetic tape material inside the plastic housing and to avoid storing them in damp conditions, or near magnetic items that could corrupt the stored data. Purpose-made plastic storage boxes available in PC stores are the best means of protecting them. The discs themselves have a small plastic slide in the bottom right hand corner. If you slide this to reveal a small square hole the disc will be protected from erasure. If you want to record more information on it then slide the plastic shutter up to cover the hole.

Sometimes the discs will have the word 'formatted' written on the box. This means that the magnetic disc material has been set up to be able to record data. If the discs are not formatted then you will need to do the following. Take an unformatted floppy disc and note the density marking on it (for example 'double density') and insert it into the disc drive bay. Click on the 'my computer' icon, which will probably be on your desktop. The next window to be displayed will show a series of icons corresponding to the drives. Click on the disc drive that you want to format. Then, from the 'file' menu, click 'format'. Remember that this will erase any data on the disc. Choose the options that you want from the dialogue box, making sure that you select the correct capacity. Then click 'start'. Do not be tempted to format your hard drive. You will lose everything on it. The rule is if you are unsure then do not do it – ask for advice and consult the help files.

Having prepared a disc, the next step is to open the word processing application and create a file.

Getting started

Open up the word processing application either from an icon on your desktop or via 'start'/'programs'/'Microsoft Word'. In longhand this means click on 'start', then click on 'programs' and then click on 'Microsoft Word' to launch the application. Having opened it you will be viewing a window. It will have a coloured title bar, a menu bar, a toolbar and, along the base, an information bar. You will notice that if you have your desktop set up as a Web page with

windows 95 or 98 or Windows Me then the mouse can be clicked on
the start button and moved up the menu, and wherever the mouse
pointer is placed over an icon a blue highlight bar will appear and
another menu opens. Just move the mouse pointer across on to the
menu and on to the required application. Then click the mouse to
open it. Thus in two clicks you should be able to find and open an
application.

The first thing to do is to create a new file. The application might
do this for you and you will have a pane within the window that is a
blank 'page'. If not, click on the menu 'file', select 'new' and, from
the window that appears, click on 'blank document' and then click
'OK'. A new pane will open and the title bar will show something
like 'Microsoft Word document 1'.

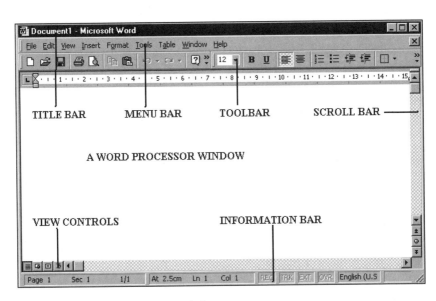

Figure 4.1 Word processor image window.

Different ways to view a window

There are different ways to view the window. The controls are found
both in the bar at the bottom of the window and also in the 'view'
menu. To change the view selection, click 'view' and the selection
desired from the drop-down menu. Alternatively, click on the view
buttons at the bottom of the window.

- *Normal view* is the best view for typing and formatting text. It simplifies the layout to facilitate typing and editing.
- *Page layout view* allows you to see how the page will be laid out for printing and is useful for viewing headers and footers and margins.
- *Print preview* displays multiple pages for your preview prior to printing out. It allows you to check the overall layout and formatting of the document. Using this view will prevent the waste of time and paper that occurs when you print copies that subsequently need to be amended.
- *Outline view* allows you to see the structure of a document, move copy and reorganize text. It allows you to see the layout of the document and to collapse a document to see just the main headings or to expand it to read the full text.
- *Master document view* allows you to manage long documents and multiple documents. It can be used to group several documents into one master document. Changes can then be made without having to open each of the individual documents.
- *Full screen view* allows you to view the document on the full screen and hide the windows tool bars.

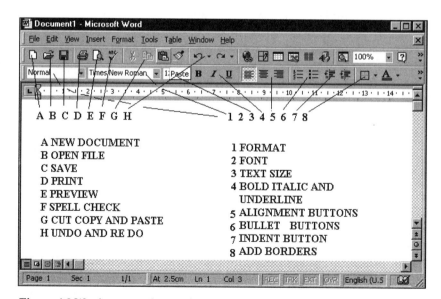

Figure 4.2 Word processor buttons image.

Naming the document

To give your document a name click 'file'/'save as' and type a name in the field labelled 'file name'. In the 'save as type' field you can select different file types but it will automatically select the one matching the application you are working with. When you have named the file, click 'save' and the blue title bar at the top of the window will display the new title. You will have noticed that the 'save as' dialogue box also has a 'save in' field where you can make a drive selection – for example the 'A' drive. Your file will be saved to whichever drive selection you make. If you right click on the small arrows at the edge of each field a small help information box should appear providing some information about the save parameter.

Using the toolbars

Having created a file and named it, the next stage is to process the text that you produce. We now discuss how to use the menu and the toolbar commands most commonly used when processing text. This is not an exhaustive study of word processing but it is intended to be sufficient to get you started so that you can create professional documents.

The toolbars can be displayed or hidden by making selection in the menu 'view'/'toolbars' menu. The following tasks that can be undertaken to format text can be achieved either by using the toolbar icons or commands in the menu bar.

Page layout

The first thing to do is to set up the page layout. To do this you click 'file'/'page setup'. You will be able to adjust the page size (for example to A4 or letter size), the margins, the paper size and paper source (for a printer), and page layout (as portrait or landscape view).

Add headers and footers and page numbers

Click on 'view'/'headers and footers' and a bar will appear on your screen that allows you to switch between the header (a box at the top of your page) or the footer (a box at the bottom of your page). You can type text into these boxes, depending on which is selected. When you click on the header and footer toolbar 'close' button the insertion point for the cursor returns to the main body of text on the page. This toolbar also has a facility to add page numbers and to format the type of number inserted.

Type in text

The cursor, as previously mentioned, will appear as a 'blinking' bar on the page. Wherever you click the mouse pointer the cursor will be positioned there so that you can go to a paragraph and edit text. The backspace key on the keyboard will delete text to the left of the cursor. The delete key on the keyboard will delete text to the right of the cursor.

Move text using 'cut', 'copy' and 'paste'

To move text, you have to select it by clicking and dragging the cursor across it so that it is highlighted. You can then click the file menu 'edit'/'copy' or right click the mouse and select 'copy'. Wherever you place the cursor and select either 'edit'/'paste' or the button 'paste', the text will be inserted. The same principle applies for the 'cut' and 'paste' commands except that 'cut' removes the selected portion of text.

Undo previous commands

If you make a mistake you can always undo the last one or more steps. To do this all you need do is click on 'edit'/'undo typing', or click on the 'undo' button. You will probably be able to undo the last six steps, depending on the version of the software that you are using.

Redo commands

The 'redo' command acts in the opposite direction to the undo 'command'. Again, it is found in the 'edit'/'redo typing' or the 'redo' button. The 'redo' function will operate only if you have undone some steps and want to retrieve a previous stage of text formatting.

Justify text

Text can be aligned to the right, left, centre or be justified where the margins appear as neat straight lines. You can do this by

- selecting a paragraph and clicking on the required alignment button

- selecting all the text and aligning all paragraphs at once
- placing the cursor at the start of a single paragraph and just setting the alignment for that one.

Remember that a paragraph is created every time that you press the 'enter' ('return') key on the keyboard. If you click on the 'paragraph marker' button you will be able to view all the spaces and paragraphs on your page.

Add columns

You can add columns to a page by using 'format'/'columns' or the 'columns' button on the standard toolbar. These can be altered in size and the number required per page.

Add bullets

A bullet is a dot placed at the start of a line of text to make it stand out, as in the section 'Justify text', above. Some software permits different choices of how the bullet is displayed such as a box, pencil or some other shape. To insert a bullet, select the paragraphs required and click on either the 'format'/'bullets and numbering' menu or on the bullet button on the 'format' toolbar.

Add numbers

You can insert numbers at the start of paragraphs in the same way that you can insert bullets. To remove numbers or bullets just place the cursor at the paragraph to be altered and click on the number button. They will then be removed.

Zooming

The standard tool bar has a zoom control that allows you to select pre-set sizes for the image of the page on your screen, or to type in a percentage size to view your pages. Some versions will also provide the options of 'page width', 'text width', 'whole page' and 'two pages'.

Increase and decrease text indents

Text can be moved as a block to the right or to the left. This is called *indenting* and is either 'increased' (moved to the right) or 'decreased' (moved back to the left). To do this, place the cursor at the paragraph to be indented and click on the 'increase indent' button. To undo the action click on the 'decrease indent' button. You can perform this action on more than one paragraph at a time by preselecting the required number of paragraphs.

Format the paragraphs.

The paragraphs can be adjusted in several ways. This includes alignment, indents, spacing and line and page breaks. If you select 'format'/'paragraphs' you will be able to view the options that can be selected and the range of individual options (usually via a drop-down menu next to the given field) that are available. This window also has an option to adjust the 'tab' settings. You will notice that, when you type in text, the 'tab' button on the keyboard (on the left-hand side with a double arrow on it) will move the text a set distance each time it is pressed. That distance can be set to match your requirements.

Select the font

The font is the script in which the text is written. There are many fonts, such as Times New Roman and Arial. To alter the font you can choose 'format'/'font' and make your selections. Alternatively, if you wish to alter the font in the text, select the required portion and click on the font field in the formatting bar. A drop-down menu at the edge of that field will provide you with a list of fonts. Just click on the one required and the text will appear in that font. Remember that if you are printing your work some fonts will use more ink. Arial and Times New Roman are popular fonts for essay and assignment submissions.

Select the text size

You can click on the font size and alter the size of the selected text in the same manner that you select a font using the formatting tool bar. This is also available through 'format'/'font'.

Bold, italic and underline

Three buttons on the format tool bar will permit these options. Just select the required text and click on the buttons as required.

Remember that if you press the 'return' or 'enter' keys at the end of any text containing these selections the next paragraph will also have them. If you do not require this in subsequent paragraphs, deselect the buttons at the appropriate place.

Add lines and boxes

Text can be selected and the 'borders' button on the format tool bar can be used to add complete or part borders. The same functions are to be found in the menu 'format'/'borders and shading'. There is also an option to add a horizontal line across the page.

Creating shortcut icons

Icons are the start buttons of applications. They are often placed on desktops for ease of access. It is possible to create a copy of an icon and drag it to the task bar so that it is in a handy place whenever you want to use it. To do this go to the icon, such as the Windows Explorer icon, which is found in 'start'/'programs', then right click on the icon and select 'copy' from the popup menu options. Next, right click somewhere on an empty part of your desktop and click on 'paste' in the pop up menu. The copied icon will appear. All you have left to do is to click and drag the icon over the task bar and release the mouse button. The icon should now appear in the task bar. If you then right click on an empty part of the task bar and from the popup menu select 'view' and then 'large', the icons will become easier to see.

So far you have been shown how to launch the word processing application and then to create a file, type and format text. The importance of file management will now be discussed.

File management

Some anecdotes follow that illustrate the importance of file management. A research assistant was compiling a database using a university network software. After about two-and-a-half hours of meticulous work the university system server, to which the computer terminal was linked, suddenly 'crashed'. 'Crashing' is a slang term for when the system suddenly stops working. This is usually evidenced by the screen 'freezing' and not responding to mouse or keyboard commands. The work was lost and the database had to be set up again. Could this have been foreseen and could anything have been done to avoid losing the work?

In fact the problem could have been avoided by setting up an auto-save function on the computer and backing up the work to a floppy disc at regular intervals.

A PhD student who had passed an important oral examination was required to make some minor but essential corrections to his thesis text by a set date. The work was stored on a university network and also on floppy discs. On the day when the work had to be completed before sending the thesis to a publisher for binding, the university system 'crashed' and was to be unavailable for two days. No problem, the student thought: the floppy discs have a copy of the whole thesis. However, when using a stand-alone PC the discs could not be read. A message screen reported that the data were corrupted.

In this case, the student's file management was thorough but he had not recently checked his discs for viruses. Networks are common sources of virus infection and their effects vary. Some, for example, stop you saving a file in the same name; others refuse access to your file at all. The solution is to virus-check the discs and 'clean' them. The data are then accessible.

There is always the chance that floppy discs will corrupt after a period of time. This is affected by the way they are stored. Even if they are virus free they might still cause problems if relied on for long-term storage. The use of server space on a network or provided by an Internet service provider (ISP) could be a good place to store data. However, you will need to be sure that it cannot be accessed by anyone else. Think of a server as a large-capacity computer on which you have a designated amount of data storage space.

The more experience you gain in using information technology the more you come across scare stories about the misfortunes of others. One recent story concerned an experienced academic who had his computer stolen. It contained research data that he had input painstakingly over many months, but that he had not backed up. Apart from the loss of valuable data, this also raised issues of security of data and confidentiality.

Another incident was at a health centre where a public health officer was working on his computer and one of the domestic staff unplugged it to use a vacuum cleaner. The result was the permanent loss of several years' immunization data on the local population.

Information gathering for evidence-based practice and other related research work will inevitably accrue large amounts of data that you will need both to analyse and synthesize into your dissertation or report. When you have made several revisions to a draft paper, it is a sudden crisis if all that hard work is lost because you have not kept copies of it. Computers can and do crash; university networks can suddenly fail and viruses can corrupt your data. It is essential, therefore, to back up your files regularly.

Creating and finding files

To create a file you can either click 'file'/'new' and follow the on-screen options, or you can click on the 'new' blank document icon on the toolbar. A blank page will appear in the word-processing window and the text insertion point (the 'blinking' cursor) will appear, usually in the top left-hand corner of the page.

To find a file previously saved on your computer or on a floppy disc you can use one of the following:

• the 'find file' explorer application
• the 'file open' menu command in a window
• the Windows Explorer browser.

Using the 'find file' explorer application

There is a 'find file' application located in the menu when you click on the start button of the task bar. If you click on 'find' and then 'files or folders' a window will open allowing you to search for the file either by drive, name, date, size or text. If you are working with a floppy disc just click on the 'A' drive and click the 'find now' button to list all the files on the floppy disc.

You will also notice that there are tabs for 'name and location', 'date' and 'advanced'. These give extra parameters to the search for a specific file. The browse button will also provide you with a range of options where you wish to commence the search. Once you see the file you are seeking then you can click on 'stop' to cease the search.

Using the 'file open' command in a word processing program

When working with a word processing application such as Word for Windows 97 you can click on the menu command word 'file' and from the drop-down menu select 'open'.

This will open up a dialogue box similar to the search for files box in the previous example. A drop-down menu box asks where you want to look for the file and other search parameters are positioned at the base of the box: 'file name', 'file type', 'text' or 'property' and 'last modified'. The file name is whatever you have chosen; the file type is the type of format the file is saved as.

The dialogue box has some small buttons along the top to select different aspects of files. These are 'list', 'details', 'properties' and 'preview'.

If you have selected the 'preview' view option for the dialogue box then, when you click on the 'find now' button, you will see the file displayed in the small square on the right-hand side. You can quickly scroll down to check whether it is the file you require. If it is, all you have to do is to click on 'open' and the file will open up in the appropriate application.

Using the Windows Explorer application

A third way of searching for files is to use the windows explorer application that is located on the program's file section. To find this click on the 'start' button then on 'programs' and then scroll down the programs until you find the Explorer icon. This opens a browser window and allows you to click on a folder on the left-hand side. This then displays the contents of that folder on the right-hand side. You can then open a file by clicking on it.

How to save your work

You will notice that the menu bar has 'file' command. Click on this and there will be a number of save options listed in the drop-down menu. If you have created a file, the first time that you try to save it, you will be prompted to give it a name and designate a location in which to save it.

'File'/'save' and 'file'/'save as'

If you click on 'file'/'save as', a dialogue box will open asking for options about saving the document. Basically you have to decide where you want to save it, then you will need to give it a file name and then save it as a particular file type. In this example it is being saved in 'C', with the file name 'My file' (click on the white space next to file name and type in what you want to call it) and the file type is Word document. This should autoselect, reflecting the application with which you are working.

Next click 'OK' and the file will be saved; the title bar of the window will now display the file name you chose.

The next time you want to save the file that you are working in, all you have to do is click on 'file'/'save'. The 'save' button on the toolbar (an icon of a floppy disc) will save the active document with its current filename, location and format.

'File'/'save all' command

You can save all open documents at the same time by clicking 'file'/'save all'. All open documents and templates are saved at the same time. If any open documents have not been previously saved then the 'save as' dialogue box is displayed so that you can name them. You can save a copy of the active document with a different name or in a different location. You can save a document in another file format. For example, you can save a Word document in a file format that can be read by earlier versions of Word or save in an HTML Web page format.

You can open a document created in a different file format, work on it in Word, and then save it in its original format. For example, you can open a Word Perfect document, edit it in Word, and then save it in either Word or Word Perfect format.

Automatic save

You can set up Word to save your work automatically at a specified interval. Click 'file'/'save as'. Next click 'options' and select the 'automatic save every . . .' check box. In the 'minutes' box enter the interval at which you want Word to save documents. When you finish setting the 'save' parameters click 'OK' to set them and return to the previous window and save the document.

Documents that are saved automatically are stored in a special format and location until you save them. When you restart Word after a power failure or other problem that occurred before you saved your work, Word opens all automatically saved documents so that you can save them.

Keep the previous version of a document when I save

This can be useful in case you want to use a previous version of text or to review the changes that you have included in the most recent version. To achieve this, do the following: on the menu, click 'file'/'save as', then click 'options', select the 'always create backup copy' check box. Click 'OK'. Click 'save'.

Viruses and virus checkers

What is a virus?

A computer virus is a program designed to replicate and spread on its own, preferably without a user's knowledge. Computer viruses spread by attaching themselves to another program, such as word processing or spreadsheet programs, or to the boot sector of a diskette. When an infected file is executed or the computer is started from an infected disc, the virus itself is executed. Often, it stays in memory, waiting to infect the next program that is run or the next disk that is accessed. Many viruses perform trigger events; for example, they might display a message on a certain date or delete files after the infected program is run a certain number of times. While some of these trigger events are benign, others can be very costly and cause significant damage.

Major sources of infection are e-mail attachments and the use of removable discs. Infection occurs most often when documents are sent as e-mail attachments, when discs that are already infected are used, or when files are copied on to other computers. The rise in Internet use is paralleled by an increase in Internet-borne malicious code carried by Microsoft ActiveX controls and Sun Microsystems Java applets. It is possible for virus writers to use ActiveX and possibly Java to introduce viruses, worms and Trojan horses on to a Web-surfer's computer, turning Web pages into virus carriers. By simply surfing the Web, users could expose their computer to viruses spread via ActiveX controls, without downloading files or even reading e-mail attachments. The virus writers could then use the virus to access RAM, corrupt files, and access files on computers attached via a local area network (LAN), among other things.

We live in a world with some malicious software authors, but why do people develop virus programs to damage other people's work? Some people like to hack into other computer users' private files; some have grievances against former employers, or even against large software companies. Whoever they are, they can create problems for other computer users. Anything you load on to your machine might contain a virus. Just as contact with other people can spread disease, so contact with other computers can spread electronic viruses. This is why organizations often have policy statements prohibiting the loading of your own software on to their systems without prior permission. There are different types of virus that act in different ways. The main point to emphasize is the need to have virus checker software and to use it to check your machine drives and your discs regularly. Anti-virus software will detect known viruses and deal with them. Some software even allows you to 'quarantine' the virus and send it to the software company to identify and provide a remedy.

It is important to

- obtain anti-virus software, which will almost certainly be part of a network system
- find the program in 'start'/'programs' and open up the virus control window, and
- review the checking options open to you, such as setting parameters to run a check every time that the machine is booted up.

You can also open the checker, select a drive and run a check on the disc in that drive. Remember that a virus checker is only as good as the last installed update of known viruses. Most companies will provide you with a link to their Web sites so that the latest virus information can be downloaded on to your machine.

I do emphasize the need to conduct checks at frequent intervals. It is really only necessary to know what to do so that your files are virus free rather than having to understand how the checker works. You will soon notice the presence of a virus, for example when commands do not work as they should.

Virus terminology

You might encounter these terms:

- A *Trojan horse* is often designed to cause damage or do something malicious to a system, but is disguised as something useful. Unlike viruses, these do not make copies of themselves.
- *Worms* are like viruses in that they do replicate themselves. They are programs that are designed to copy themselves from one computer to another, infecting an entire system.
- Viruses are either *benign* or *malignant*. A benign virus might simply display a message at a given time or slows down the operation of the computer. A malignant virus causes damage to a computer system, such as corrupting files or destroying data.
- A *virus hoax* is an e-mail that is intended to scare people about a non-existent virus threat. Users often forward these alerts thinking they are doing a service to their fellow workers. This is time wasting and tends to act as a chain letter clogging up e-mail systems. There are pages available on the Internet dedicated to informing you about hoaxes through the sites listed in the next paragraph.

Further information about viruses

If you wish to know more about computer viruses then you can find a brief introduction at http://www.symantec.com/. Further information about anti-virus software can be obtained either from the information packs purchased with software from high-street stores or at the following web sites: http://www.symantec.com/ (Norton anti-virus software); http://www.mcafee.com/ (McAfee anti-virus software); http://www.drsolomon.com/ (Dr Solomon's anti-virus software).

Exercises

Create a new file in a word processing application and give that file a name by using one of the 'save' options such as 'file'/'save as'. Copy the following six paragraphs of text and title.

Word processing text example

A PhD student who had passed an important oral examination was required to make some minor but essential corrections to his thesis text by a set date. The work was stored on a university network and also on floppy discs. On the day when the work had to be completed before sending the thesis to a publisher for binding, the university system 'crashed' and was to be unavailable for two days. No problem, the student thought: the floppy discs have a copy of the whole thesis. However, when using a stand-alone PC the discs could not be read. A message screen reported that the data were corrupted.

In this case, the student's file management was thorough but he had not recently checked his discs for viruses. Networks are common sources of virus infection and their effects vary. Some, for example, stop you saving a file in the same name; others refuse access to your file at all. The solution is to virus-check the discs and 'clean' them. The data are then accessible.

There is always the chance that floppy discs will corrupt after a period of time. This is affected by the way they are stored. Even if they are virus free they might still cause problems if relied on for long-term storage. The use of server space on a network or provided by an Internet service provider (ISP) could be a good place to store data. However, you will need to be sure that it cannot be accessed by anyone else. Think of a server as a large-capacity computer on which you have a designated amount of data storage space.

The more experience you gain in using information technology the more you come across scare stories about the misfortunes of others. One recent story concerned an experienced academic who had his computer stolen. It contained research data that he had input painstakingly over many months, but that he had not backed up. Apart from the loss of valuable data, this also raised issues of security of data and confidentiality.

Another incident was at a health centre where a public health officer was working on his computer and one of the domestic staff unplugged it to use a vacuum cleaner. The result was the permanent loss of several years' immunization data on the local population.

Information gathering for evidence-based practice and other related research work will inevitably accrue large amounts of data that you will need both to analyse and synthesize into your dissertation or report. When you have made several revisions to a draft paper, it is a sudden crisis if all that hard work is lost because you have not kept copies of it. Computers can and do crash; university networks can suddenly fail and viruses can corrupt your data. It is essential, therefore, to back up your files regularly!

Now complete the following tasks to practise using some of the word processor functions. Insert a page break at the end of the text. Select and copy all of that text and insert it after the page break. You will now have two pages of identical text. You will format the second page and be able to see the difference from the first page when you have finished.

1. Select the new page and adjust the right margin size to 4 cm.
2. Add headers and footers – put in a title and date for example, and page numbers.
3. Select the first paragraph and justify the text.
4. Select the second paragraph and right align the text.
5. Select the third paragraph and left align the text
6. Select the fourth paragraph and centre the text
7. Select paragraphs five and six and add bullets using the bullet button.
8. Select the first four paragraphs and add numbers using the numbering icon.
9. Alter the view size of the page using the zoom function on the standard toolbar.
10. Select the last two paragraphs and indent them using the increase indent button.
11. Select the first two paragraphs and title, and alter the font to Arial.
12. Select the remainder of the text and make the font Times New Roman.
13. Select the title and alter the font size to 14 point.
14. Select all the rest of the text and make the font size 10 point.
15. Make the title bold in italics and underlined.
16. Insert a border around each of the last two paragraphs.

Other places where you can find help with word processing

Your local college or university might offer computer literacy courses in particular those leading to a recognized qualification such as the CLAIT (Computer Literacy and Information Technology) certificate.

Chapter 5
The Internet and
Internet browser

The history of the Internet and the WWW

The Internet was created on 2 January 1969 when US computer scientists began researching computer networking. This research was funded by the Advanced Research Projects Agency (ARPA), which gave the Internet its first name, the ARPANET. The ARPANET was used to test the use of packet-switched networks, which are computer networks that transfer information in the form of little packets that move independently of each other through various networks until they reach their final destination.

The US Department of Defense Advanced Research Projects Agency originally developed the Internet to be a military communication system that could survive a nuclear war. Despite its military background it was used by the National Science Foundation (NSF) in the US academic community to create a research support system. It became a means of instant communications between computer researchers across the US. In 1983, the ARPANET was reserved for civilian use, while MILNET was created for military use. Communications between the two networks was possible, and this network became known as the 'Internet'.

The research behind the technology was developed at CERN. This is the European Laboratory for Particle Physics, the world's largest particle physics centre. Founded in 1954, the laboratory was one of Europe's first joint ventures, and is located on the outskirts of Geneva. From the original 12 signatories of the CERN convention, membership now includes 19 member states. For more information about this laboratory and its work studying the nature of matter visit its Web site at the following Internet address (details of how to use an Internet address follow): http//www.cern.ch/Public/.

As the Internet grew during the 1980s, more networks were formed to serve various communities and organizations. In 1986, the National Science Foundation (NSF) again connected researchers and organizations with the NSFNET, which consisted of five super-computer systems. During this time many other nations began developing their own versions of the NSFNET. All of these networks are now interconnected to form the significantly more powerful Internet that we know today. Connections to the Internet are usually by telephone or fibre optic cable, but can be via satellite and wireless application protocol devices such as mobile telephones.

The Internet differs from a *local area network* (LAN), which is a system consisting of one server and many clients, and clients access information stored on a server. An example of a LAN is an office with three computers connected to each other but not to any other network. There is no central server on the Internet. Instead, there are thousands of host machines that can both send and receive information to and from other hosts. In this way, each host on the Internet behaves as both a server and a client.

The actual physical network of the Internet consists of a massive web of transmission lines, each line capable of transferring a specified amount of data (this limitation is called bandwidth). This 'web' of transmission lines is designed so that information from any site can reach its destination using any of thousands of different possible paths. When information is sent over this network, it is split into tiny packets. Each packet of information travels to its destination using a different route. When all of the packets reach their destination, the packets are regrouped to form the original piece of information. If one or more of the packets doesn't successfully make its destination, the receiving site simply asks for another copy of those packets.

What use is it to me?

The Internet offers different things to each individual. Personal experience of using it will soon reveal both some of its benefits and some of its limitations as a means of accessing information. Some of the benefits include access to pages of information and databases on thousands of topics, Web-based communication – such as instant messaging, chat rooms, e-mail and multimedia information (music, video). Another service is Usenet, a system of newsgroups, each of which is dedicated to a specific topic of interest. People worldwide can post to and read messages from Usenet newsgroups almost instantaneously.

The World Wide Web (WWW or 'Web')

The World Wide Web, or simply the Web, has transformed the task of finding information on the Internet from a difficult to a simple one. Technically speaking, the Web is an information retrieval system consisting of an international network of computers that are all interconnected using hypertext links (described in detail in the next section). The Web also features multimedia abilities. Multimedia refers to the fact that, in addition to text, the Web uses graphics, audio, and video.

Hypertext is what makes the Web so valuable. But what is it? Hypertext is simply a type of document (found on the Web) that contains links (called hyperlinks) that point your Web browser to another resource on the Internet. A hyperlink can be in the form of a word, several words, or even an image. When you select a hyperlink with your Web browser (usually by clicking the link with your mouse), your Web browser automatically loads whatever the selected link indicates. A link such as this would differ from rest of the document either by being underlined, coloured, or highlighted, depending on your Web browser. Often, more than one of these methods is used to distinguish hyperlinks. When visited (by clicking on a link) the colour of the hypertext often changes.

When searching you can move quickly through a series of documents following keywords or links to other related material. The Web can be used as a virtual library that can bring thousands of documents, on just about any subject, to the monitor of any Internet user within seconds. If you were using a paper-based library then this would entail getting other books off shelves and thumbing through them to find the appropriate related material. Thus what once took a lot of time can now be accomplished at the click of a mouse, although it remains limited to the resources actually available in electronic form.

Today, whilst there are attempts to set standards for using the Internet there is no one particular group in charge of it. There is no single government or commercial organization running the Internet and there are no official rules that govern its use. Instead, the

Internet is kept up and running by the collective efforts of every organization with a computer or network connected to the Internet, each forming a vital part of the Internet infrastructure. Overall, the Internet is a mixture of commercial, political, academic and personal interests and, as such, many of the sites reflect these user groups. Governments may attempt to introduce regulation and censorship but it is difficult for them to police. The Internet does not have geographical boundaries. It can link people with similar interests. It allows access to countless resources rather like a huge virtual library of information. It allows communication with others even when they are not using their computer. It currently allows freedom of speech.

A few groups provide many of the information services on the Internet. The Information Sciences Institute (ISI) does much of the standardization and allocation work for the Internet, acting as the Internet Assigned Numbers Authority (IANA). SRI International provides the principal information services for the Internet by operating the Network Information Center (NIC).

Its drawbacks are that it can be vulnerable to hackers who try to look at private information stored electronically. It can carry viruses to your computer. It is fast and yet connections can be slow depending upon the demands placed on various servers. However, once you are able to use *search engines* (information-finding aids) on the Internet then you will be able to retrieve a wealth of technical information about almost any subject that you care to name.

The Internet provides several basic services. Many of these are available through *Internet service providers* (ISPs) who offer free access and the necessary software to get online. The services include: electronic mail (e-mail); newsgroups; mailing lists; access to files on remote computers; online database searching. Other services include video conferencing, voice conferencing, multimedia broadcasts and Internet radio.

To go online you will need communications software, which is often provided free by ISPs, and a modem, which converts the information from your computer into a form that can be transmitted along a cable. The purpose of this section is to give you an insight into connecting to the Internet, without dwelling on technicality. Modern computer packages come with both the hardware and software as a standard package and so you shouldn't have to know much more than following the on-screen directions and make sure that modem cables are connected.

What is a modem?

A modem is a device that allows two computers to communicate over a standard phone line. This is accomplished by changing the digital information of a computer (which is stored as a series of 0s and 1s known as the binary code) into a tone, or frequency, that can be sent over the phone to another modem. The receiving modem will then change the sent tones back to digital information, which can be understood by the receiving computer. This process gives the modem its name, derived from the two words 'modulate' and 'demodulate', which accurately describe the two primary functions of a modem.

Modems can be fitted inside the computer or connected to it externally using a cable. External modems are slightly more expensive than internal ones.

What is ISDN?

An Integrated Services Digital Network (ISDN) telephone line transfers pure digital information, unlike a standard phone line that was designed solely for voice (analogue) communications. Integrated Services Digital Network lines can transfer data at 128 Kbps, many times faster than current modems.

The Internet can now be accessed by telephone cable, digital cable and more recently by using a wireless application protocol (WAP) device. The trend for the future will probably be to move to wireless devices, but the cable-linked computer is still likely to be predominant in the short to medium term.

To use an ISDN line to connect to the Internet check out the best deals on offer with the different telecommunications companies. The competition between these companies means that new deals are frequently marketed and so to suggest one here it would soon be out-of-date information.

Communications software

Communications software allows your computer to communicate with other computers connected to the Internet. This can be done only by using software that 'speaks' the language of the Internet. This language is called TCP/IP, which stands for Transmission Control Protocol/Internet Protocol. It is the standard language of the Internet, and your computer, like every other computer connected to the Internet, must have some sort of TCP/IP 'translator'. This is where your TCP/IP communications software comes in. In most cases your TCP/IP software is also used to connect with your Internet provider (in other words, to dial their modem) and establish a connection. It is because of this feature that TCP/IP software is often referred to as a 'TCP dialler'.

You can obtain this software from ISPs or on free CD ROM sold with computer magazines or given away in retail stores. Often it comes as part of a preloaded package when you buy a computer. If you get a free CD ROM and insert it in your CD disc drive it more often than not will auto-run and an information screen will appear on the monitor screen with instructions to follow a series of steps to set up an Internet account that gives you e-mail addresses, space on a server to post your own Web page and a browser to be able to view web pages. Often there are help files to guide you through creating a Web page. You can also find online services such as Microsoft Network Hotmail, which gives a free mail account, your own web page and much more besides. The Internet addresses for some free online services such as e-mail and Web pages include http://www.microsoft.com/(Microsoft Hotmail) and http://www.freeserve.net/(Freeserve).

Internet service providers (ISPs)

An Internet service provider is simply a company that provides Internet access to the public. Internet service provider access charges vary, so you are advised to check out how their service compares before you make a selection. These are increasingly becoming free services but their telephone helpline charges for technical support might carry a high tariff (for example, you might have to call a premium rate number).

An ISP operates computers that are connected directly to the Internet. Customers connect to these computers and either connect directly to the Internet or use software on the ISP's computers to access the Internet. Although there are a few national ISPs, most ISPs are regional and might be restricted to a single city or geographical region. Computer magazines frequently compare the services and rank the ISPs. There are some things that the potential customer should ask an ISP before purchasing an account. It is necessary to know that you can go online whenever you dial up a connection or whether the ISP is known for having so many customers that there is an engaged tone every time you try to connect. Some ISPs that require you to transfer your telephone account to them and offer free online time (no telephone bill) might disconnect you (called *timing out*) after a set period. Some ISPs have a set per minute online charge that is designed to undercut competitors in the communications field. Having said that, you can redirect your telephone charging through another company without having to transfer your telephone line rental and phone rental billing.

How to connect to the Internet

The *Internet connection wizard* provides you with a step-by-step guide on how to connect to the Internet. For new Internet users, the Internet connection wizard creates an Internet connection for you, and then displays a list of Internet service providers (ISPs) and information about their services. You can sign up for a new account by clicking an ISP in the list. To run the wizard click on 'tools'/'Internet options'/'connections'/'set up' and follow the on-screen instructions.

The Internet browser

The *browser* is the window that you use to view pages on the Internet. It is a piece of computer software that views Web pages. In addition to simply downloading and displaying the textual information of a Web page, most Web browsers automatically display images too. Web browsers are also capable of accessing gopher directories, downloading FTP files, and sending e-mail. It is this versatility that makes Web browsers so useful when using the Internet. With a single application, you can now access practically everything on the Net – all with a few clicks of a mouse.

Understanding the browser

This section guides you through some of the key functions of the browser. It might help if you have the computer booted up and launch the browser by clicking on the intenet icon. The example used will be the Microsoft Internet Explorer. Other browsers will have the same general principles, although sometimes they use different words for the same idea, such as 'bookmarks' instead of 'favorites' for the facility for saving Web page addresses. Nevertheless, generally speaking, once you learn how to use one browser you will be able to navigate using others.

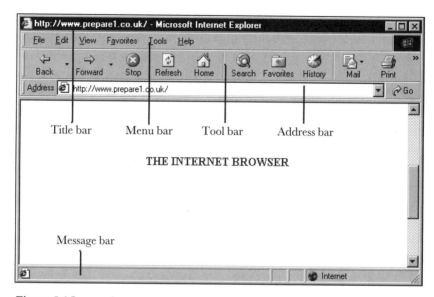

Figure 5.1 Internet browser.

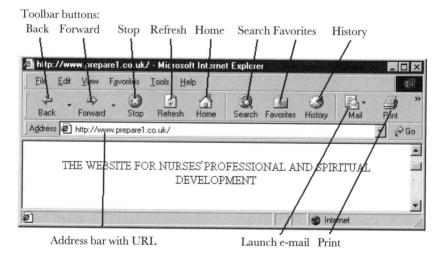

Figure 5.2 Browser controls.

The general layout of the browser is that it is a window and has along the top of it a dark blue title bar that will display the heading of the Web page you are viewing.

Next there are a series of grey bars, the first being the menu bar, then the toolbar, an address bar, the viewing window itself displaying the Web page and, along the bottom of the window, a status bar. Each of these will be discussed in turn.

The purpose of understanding the browser is to be able to adjust the view of it to suit your preferences and to be able to operate it so that you can locate information on the Internet.

The title bar has the same format as a word-processing window with small buttons on the right hand side to minimize, restore and close the browser window. The title of the Web page that you are viewing will be displayed in this title bar.

The menu bar is also in the same format as the word processing window. In the Microsoft example being used the menus are 'file', 'edit', 'view', 'favorites', 'tools' and 'help'.

The next bar is the address bar. This has a field that displays the Internet address of a page (called a URL) and a button marked 'go'.

The grey bar along the base of the browser window is the status bar. This displays information about what the browser is doing. It will show the address of hyperlink pages as you pass your mouse pointer over them, and also a message that it is opening the page if you click on the link. In addition the bar will display a blue line showing the progress in opening a Web page. Small icons will also be displayed in this bar including a globe that, when you click on it, will open up a utility permitting you to adjust the browser's Internet security properties. A padlock will also be displayed at times indicating that you are accessing a secure site that claims to be safe when transmitting information such as credit card details.

The menu bar

If you click on the menus you will see that some of their contents are similar to those of a word processor menu window.

The 'file' menu

The 'file open' command launches a dialogue box that allows you to type in an Internet address and then, when you click on the 'OK' button, finds the required Web page.

The 'work offline' command, when clicked, will let you work offline (indicated by a tick next to the command). When clicked again it places you back online. An icon will appear in the status bar with a cross on it to indicate that you are working offline. If you hover the mouse pointer over this icon a text message will appear to tell you that you are working offline and that, to connect, you have to click 'work online' in the file menu.

The view menu

This menu allows you to view a range of toolbars. Clicking on each word will place a tick next to each one and place it in view. Reversing the action will remove each one. You can also customize the toolbar by adding a range of different icons found in the dialogue box that appears when you click on the menu word 'view'/'toolbars'/ 'customize'.

Status bar

Clicking on this will switch the view on or off.

Explorer bar

This relates to three toolbar icons – 'search', 'history' and 'favorites'. Clicking on each one will split the main browser window.

'Search' displays a search engine facility to find things on the Internet (discussed in the chapter on information searching strategies). 'Favorites' displays Web pages and folders that you have stored and organized according to your preferences. This is also discussed in the chapter on information searching strategies. 'History' displays all the Web pages that you have previously visited in the past few months. To do this click on the menu 'tools'/'Internet options'. A tab file screen will appear that informs you that the history folder contains links to pages you have visited for quick access to recently viewed pages. There is a box to adjust a figure setting up to the past 99 days. What you see in the history pane is a list of folders and pages contained within them. You can click on the folder and a given page and the browser will start to open that page.

The command 'text size' permits you to alter the size of text viewed in the browser window on a Web page through five options, from largest to smallest.

'Full screen' will enlarge the browser to full screen size. To revert to the previous view option just click on the 'restore' icon in the top right corner if the address bar. The other screen items such as the task bar will be hidden. If you need to view the task bar then place the mouse pointer at the bottom of the screen and the task bar should pop up into view.

Favorites

This is a command that permits you to save – and categorize in folders – Web pages of interest that you wish to find again easily. Once a page has been stored in 'favorites' you just click on the menu and find the folder and page, and clicking on it will open up that page.

Tools

This menu includes an e-mail facility and an 'Internet options' control tab file box. E-mail will be discussed in a subsequent chapter. The 'Internet options' control tab file box, as mentioned earlier, allows you to adjust various settings. These are 'general'; 'security'; 'content'; 'connections'; 'programs' and 'advanced'.

General

This allows you to type in an address that sets up the home page that will display whenever you first launch the browser. You can also set up the parameters of temporary Internet files that your computer will create whenever you visit a page. Leave this as the default setting unless you find that your computer is running short on memory storage space, in which case you could click on 'delete files' or adjust the maximum memory that you want to allocate to these files. The third option on this tab is 'history' and has already been mentioned.

Security settings

These allow you to set parameters for designated and non-designated sites that you wish to view, and to place limitations on what you will download from each designated site. An important message that you will see occasionally is to 'ensure that cookies are enabled on you computer'. A cookie is described in the resources section. To view Web pages quickly they are usually enabled. To check the settings on your computer do the following: Click on the menu 'tools'/'Internet options' and then the tab 'security' and then on the button or the particular site (you have four choices here but most probably will select the 'Internet Web zone' rather than 'intranet', 'trusted' and 'restricted' sites. Click on the custom level button and scroll down the settings screen to find the heading 'cookies'. Make sure that the radio button is checked for 'enable cookies'. Then click on the OK button.

Content

This tab allows you to adjust the content that you wish to view on screen. It includes content, certificates and an option to record personal information. If you click on the 'content advisor' option you can set the limitations on language, nudity, sex and violence. Full details are clearly displayed and there is also a link to a rating site that provides more details about the rating of Web sites. You can even set a password protection option to prevent others, such as children, from viewing certain Web sites.

Connections

This has a utility that will guide you about how to connect to the Internet and will request some specific details if you are connecting up a PC. If you are working on a network you will not need to adjust these settings.

Programs

This tab allows you to specify the service windows automatically uses for each Internet service. Leave this as the default setting if you are new to using the Internet.

Advanced

This tab is important to you in that occasionally you will see an on-screen message that asks you to make sure that 'cookies are enabled'. Leave the settings as default unless you are certain about what you are doing, but look through the options in this tab. You will notice that there are lists of statements under the headings of 'accessibility', 'browsing', 'HTTP settings', 'Microsoft VM', 'multimedia', 'printing', 'search from the address bar' and 'security'.

One option is of particular note: printing. Make sure that the box 'print background colours and images' is not checked unless you really want all of the graphics as well as text printing. Checking this will soon use up your printer's ink cartridge.

The help menu

This contains a range of help files and sometimes an online tutorial.

The toolbar

The purpose of the toolbar is a quick shortcut to frequently used functions such as printing. The bar displays a range of buttons and these will be discussed next. You can customize what is displayed by clicking 'view'/ 'toolbars'/'customize' or by right clicking on the toolbar and selecting 'customize' from the pop-up menu. Follow the dialogue window instructions to add or remove buttons.

The principal buttons are:

- *Back button.* Click this to return to the previous page.
- *Forward button.* Click this to go to the next page in a series of pages that you have already visited. An arrow on each button reveals a drop down menu displaying previous pages visited.
- *Refresh button.* Click this to update the current page if the information does not appear or seems to be loading very slowly. It will also update old information on a page.
- *Home button.* Click this to go to your *home page* (the first page you see when you open your browser).
- *Search button.* Click this to open the 'search' bar, where you can choose a search engine service to search the Internet.
- *Favorites button.* Click this to open the 'favorites' bar, where you can store links (shortcuts) to your most frequently visited Web sites or documents.

The address bar

Type Web-page addresses (URLs) or paths to documents here. The auto-complete feature saves you typing in full addresses by displaying previously visited addresses. If you have typed in the address before a list of matches appears. If you click on the one required, the page will be retrieved. To do this click 'tools'/'Internet options'/'content tab'/ under personal information click 'auto complete' and check the boxes you want to be applied. (The options are 'Web addresses', 'forms', 'usernames' and 'passwords' on forms, 'prompt me to save passwords'.)

The status bar

The left side of the bar displays a statement about Web-page loading progress. The right side tells you the security zone that the current page is in, and shows a lock icon if you are on a secure site.

Downloading

Using the Internet safely

You can find pictures, sounds, or programs to download (install) to your computer from the Internet. When you click on a Web page that offers to download something to your hard disc it transfers files to you. These will be stored in a file, typically 'downloaded program files', which can be found by using the Windows Explorer utility in the 'start' menu or in the 'start'/'programs' folder.

Increasing the speed at which you view Web pages

When viewing Web pages you can 'turn off' graphics so that it loads faster. To do this click on 'tools'/'Internet options'/'advanced' tab. Under 'multimedia' uncheck one or more of these boxes: 'show pictures'; 'play animations'; 'play videos'; 'play sounds'. If the pictures on the current page are still visible after the check box has been 'unchecked' click on 'view'/'refresh'.

The Microsoft Internet Explorer help files also have some guidance 'tips' for Netscape navigator users.

Adding extras to the browser function: helper applications or plug-ins

There are many different file types on the Internet and no single program can read them all. This is why *helpers* and *plug-ins* are needed. A helper is a program that works beside a large program such as Microsoft Internet Explorer to do some job that it cannot do, or cannot do as well as the helper. A plug-in is a program that can seamlessly handle some file type within a main program such as Internet Explorer. These plug-ins might enable you to read files, listen to sound files, view video files and different formats of graphics. Many online articles, especially from government Web sites, are in portable document format (PDF). The sites will often have a link to the required software for downloading. Once downloaded you will be able to read these types of files.

How do you use helper programs?

Once you have downloaded and set up the browser to recognize helper programs it will automatically call upon them when required. Some recent versions of browsers will automatically configure themselves to recognize downloaded programs. There is generally no configuration needed to use a plug-in.

Common helpers and plug-ins include:

- *Adobe Acrobat Reader* is the free software helper from Adobe Systems (http://www.adobe.com/) and is used to read files in Adobe's portable document format (PDF).
- *JPEGView* is a fast, powerful image viewer helper. It can open and display images in formats including JPEG, PICT, GIF, TIFF, and BMP.

The URL – the address of a Web page

The objective of this section is for you to be able to recognize and understand what the component parts of a uniform resource locator (URL) mean. You will need to understand the importance of typing in an accurate URL address to be able to view a specific Web page.

What are URLs?

A uniform resource locator (URL) is a standard way of specifying the location of a resource available electronically. Uniform resource locators are defined by internationally agreed specifications. They make it possible to direct people and software applications to a variety of information available from a number of different Internet protocols. Most commonly, you will run into URLs when using a WWW client as that medium uses URLs to link WWW pages together. In your WWW browser's 'location' box, the item that generally starts with 'http:' is a URL. Files available over protocols besides HTTP, such as FTP and Gopher can be referenced by URLs.

A URL is like your complete mailing address: it specifies all the information necessary for someone to find the address of a specific page on a server. However, they are much more than that because URLs can refer to a variety of very different types of resources. A more fitting analogy would be a system for specifying your mailing address, your phone number, or the location of the book you just read from the public library, all in the same format.

In short, a URL is a very convenient and succinct way to direct people and applications to a file or other electronic resource. Learning how to interpret a URL will greatly assist your exploration of the Internet.

General URL syntax

All URLs follow the format:

scheme:scheme-dependent information

Examples of various schemes are 'http', 'gopher', 'ftp', and 'news'. The scheme tells you or the application using the URL the type of resource we are trying to reach and/or what mechanism to use to obtain that resource.

The scheme-dependent information is detailed below with each separate scheme. However, most schemes include two different types of information:

•   the Internet machine making the file available, and

- the 'path' to that file.

With these types of schemes we generally see the scheme separated from the Internet address of the machine with two forward slashes (//), and then the Internet address separated from the full path to the file with one slash (/). FTP, HTTP, and Gopher URLs generally appear in this fashion:

> scheme://machine.domain/full-path-of-file

As an exercise, let's look at this file's URL:

> http://www.uclan.ac.uk/

It is the address of a university home page. If typed into the 'file'/'open' dialogue box then the University of Central Lancashire homepage would be shown. The scheme for this URL is:

- http – for the hypertext transfer protocol (a protocol is a set of rules and standards that enables computers to exchange information)
- www – the page uses World Wide Web protocols
- uclan.ac.uk – this means that the Web server is at the University of Central Lancashire (Uclan)
- ac – denotes an academic institution;
- uk – denotes the country of the institution. The name of a company or institution is called a domain name and it has a range of possible suffixes. Some of them are: .co, .com, .ac, .org, and .mil.

Once at the home page for the institution then you can click on a link and you will notice that the address bar details change and a path to a particular file within that site is shown. An example of this is:

> http://www.uclan.ac.uk/library/libhom1.htm

This describes the scheme (http) and the use of the www protocol. The domain name is a university (uclan.ac.uk) and the path to the page displayed is a library Web page, and the home page of the library in particular.

Web pages use a special language known as hypertext mark up language (HTML) hence the extension on the www address.

Most URLs will appear very similar to the example given. Sometimes the browser will retrieve a site without your having to type in the 'http://' portion of the address.

Note that when using FTP, HTTP, and Gopher URLs, the 'full-path-of-file' will sometimes end in a slash. This indicates that the URL is pointing not to a specific file but a directory. In this case, the server generally returns the 'default index' of that directory. This might be just a listing of the files available within that directory, or a default file that the server automatically looks for in the directory. With HTTP servers, this default index file is generally called 'index.html', but is frequently seen as 'homepage.html', 'home.html', 'welcome.html', or 'default.html'.

More about domain names

A domain is specified by the two or three letter URL suffix that tells you what kind of site it is. For example, if you type the wrong domain, such as 'www.name.org' instead of 'www.name.co', 'www.name.com' or 'www.name.ac' the site may not be found. If you are unsure, try a logical alternative.

Each domain name has an IP address assigned to it – sometimes you will see a series of numbers appear in the status bar at the bottom of the browser window a when you are connecting to a Web site. This is the IP address but you do not need to know this, hence the usefulness of domain names that are easier to remember. They are also used because they are more permanent than IP addresses. A domain name consists of several parts: the top-level domain (TLD), the subdomain, and the host name. The TLD is the broadest part of a domain name and comes last in the domain name. The subdomain comes directly before the TLD. Any number of host names can precede the subdomain.

You will encounter many top-level domains on the Internet. Some are national and others international (and may be used by any computer on the Internet). Some examples of domains are:

.gov   – government
.edu – education
.ac – academic
.com – commercial
.mil – military
.org – non-profit organizations
.int – international organizations and Internet databases.

More detailed listings of domain names can be found at http://www.credible.com.

Using URLs

Now that you know what a WWW address looks like you can point your browser to a specific location. Such addresses appear in many types of advertising now as companies and organizations seek to establish a virtual presence as well as a physical one. It is a good idea to keep a notebook with useful addresses in, as well as in the 'book-marks' or 'favorites' folders of your browser.

There are two ways of inputting a WWW address. One is to click 'open location' and type in the address and click file 'find'. The other way is to type the address into the address bar. Note that you do have the option to hide this bar. To make it visible click on the browser menu 'view' and select 'toolbars'. You will then be able to check the items to be visible in the browser.

Hypertext, as detailed in an earlier chapter, is the section of a Web page where the mouse pointer changes from an arrow to (usually) a pointing finger. When this happens the pointer is over a hyperlink – for example text or a graphic. The message bar at the bottom of the browser will display the URL, and to go to that page just click the mouse button.

Finding a Web site when a Web address doesn't work

Sometimes you will try to follow a URL to its destination and will not meet with success. If the remote machine refuses the connection it is quite possible that the site is very busy. Many popular sites cannot be contacted during peak hours. If the file cannot be found, check how you spelled the URL to ensure that you are correctly specifying it. Try removing the file name, and referencing the directory in which the file supposedly resides. Perhaps the file was misspelled when given to you, and you might find the correct spelling in the index. If that doesn't work, maybe the file was moved, and you could try looking up the hierarchy by sequentially removing the last directory in the path listed until you come to the root directory for that site's server.

The Internet Explorer browser has a setup function that can be configured to search for the name you type in and to search for addresses that contain that name, and either suggest possible matches or automatically go to the first match. To set this up click on 'tools'/'Internet options' on the browser menu bar, then the 'advanced' tab and select the radio button display the results and go to the most likely sites. Previous versions of the Internet browser might have a statement something like this under a heading 'search when URL fails':

- If you don't want Internet Explorer to search for a similar address, click NEVER SEARCH.
- If you want Internet Explorer to ask if you want it to search when an address fails, click 'always ask'.
- If you want Internet Explorer to search without asking first, click ALWAYS SEARCH.
- If you want Internet Explorer to search for the address using a different domain, select the AUTOSCAN COMMON ROOT DOMAINS check box.

Chapter 6
Information-searching strategies using the Internet browser

Introduction

The Internet is so vast that it is important to be able to locate the information that you require efficiently. To browse the Web hoping to find what you need is akin to walking into a public library with hundreds of texts and hoping to find a particular page in a given book. It cannot be done quickly unless you are either lucky or have a methodical search strategy.

A clearly thought-out strategy involves two considerations. It is necessary, first, to try to conceptualize the field and second to know which part of the field of information you are searching in. However, the Internet is so vast that it is difficult to map it out as a whole. It is difficult to know whether or not what can be found has been found. In the days of hand searching paper-based literature you would have had to use card index systems, publications of journal indexes, and perhaps even visit or write to different locations to track down circulars, executive directives and other non-indexed 'grey' literature.

The Internet, for the purposes of this book, can be conceptualized in four main information domains:

- academic
- political
- commercial
- personal.

The search methodology suggested begins by trying to conceptualize the 'field' of information in your given topic area. The first two topic areas are likely to be of interest and offer useful content for the purposes of professional practice. The second two topic areas will tend to be leisure, non-peer reviewed, 'lay' as opposed to professional discipline-based knowledge sites. They frequently try to sell some product or service.

The sites that I have labelled 'political and academic' often contain many links to useful resources, including databases and journals. Once you find a site that is going to be visited frequently you can store the URL in the 'favorites' folder. This site might be a 'professional' resource such as a clinical information database that has its own specific search engine to search within that area alone. Soon, with a little practice, you will be finding sites relevant to your topic area and creating your own directory in the 'favorites' folder.

Searching strategies

Conceptualizing the field with broad searches

The range of information on the internet about a particular subject can be discovered by using Web directories available from a range of companies such as Microsoft Network, Lycos, Excite and Yahoo! However, these can sometimes seem to be only one step up from a lucky-dip approach to finding information on the Internet.

A *directory* is a Web page that contains headings and subheadings that you can select to view a given page. These subsequent pages are often subdirectories and offer links to a range of information within a specified area.

Directory searching can be likened to searching for a given leaf on a tree. First you have to choose the tree to get the leaf from – selecting a directory to start with. There are many directory services on the internet.

Next a heading has to be selected – this might be likened to selecting which branch to climb.

Having selected a tree (the homepage of the directory) and a branch (a main heading) now select a secondary branch off the main branch (subheadings within the main heading chosen).

Next you move from the secondary branch to a twig (a sub-subheading). At the twig you might see a cluster of leaves (pages that

you can view). You then select one of them. A real example follows
from the Microsoft Network page:

- Step 1. Chose a directory: http://www.msn.com/. This page has
  many alphabetically arranged directory-based finding aids such
  as cars, business, careers, city guides, computing and the Web
  through to sports, travel and women.
- Step 2. Just suppose that you wanted to find out about diabetes.
  You would guess that it might come under the 'health' heading of
  the main directory. Clicking on that takes you to another page:
  http://www.health.msn.com/.
- Step 3. This page has a variety of information such as a selection
  under 'Newly diagnosed? You are not alone', which has a
  heading for 'diabetes'. You could select that heading and click
  on the 'GO' button. Alternatively you could select from the
  heading 'Conditions A–Z'. This takes you to a page
  http://www.content.health.msn.com/condition_center_overview.
- Step 4. A new directory of headings is available and you look
  down the list until you find the condition about which you want to
  find information. In this case 'diabetes'. Clicking on this takes you
  to a page http://content.health.msn.com/condition_center/dia.
- Step 5. On this page there is a wealth of topic-related information
  from a small directory with 'diabetes basics' including the following: 'Overview, treatment, diagnosis, complementary therapies,
  self-care, newly diagnosed.' In addition there are 90 current articles
  about the topic. This page is akin to having found a twig with a
  number of leaves each carrying a piece of information. The search
  is completed by deciding to view information about a specific issue,
  in this case diagnosis.

To get to that place in the search has taken five steps. You might wish
to keep a record of your directory searches and write the steps as
follows:

www.msn.com/health/conditions A–Z/diabetes/diagnosis.

Another example uses a different directory for the same enquiry to
show that the same search enquiry can be carried out in different
ways:

- Step 1. Select the directory http://uk.yahoo.com/.
- Step 2. Click on the word 'health'.
- Step 3. Click on 'diseases and conditions'.
- Step 4. Look down the directory list and click on 'diabetes'.
- Step 5. Whilst you might want to find out about diagnosis there is not a specific directory heading listing this word and so you would have to try a site from the many offered such as 'A doctor's guide to the Internet – a guide to diabetes-related information and resources likely to be of interest to medical professionals and/or patients'.

You might wish to record that search in the following way:

> http://www.yahoo.com/health/diseases and conditions/diabetes/a doctor's guide.

Once again this is five steps through a directory to arrive near specific information – in this case a different range of information from that supplied by Microsoft Network.

How useful is a directory search?

Each directory, or Web guide, is a page with a list of hypertext links to other pages under that general heading that have been indexed with that site. This means that a process of selection has occurred, exercised by whoever has constructed the categories within the directory. Thus there is not a single Web directory that includes all the information on the Internet.

A directory search has the benefit, however, of allowing you to follow links within categories as you move from link to link towards some specific area of information. This is like searching in a *Yellow Pages* paper directory for a supplier of car exhausts. You would look under 'retailers', and then perhaps 'automotive retailers', then 'automotive retailers of exhausts' and finally choose one in your geographical location.

The results of a broad search might offer thousands of hits, some of which will be useful. The next task therefore is to be able to narrow a topic field down through refining the search terms.

What you will be able to gather from the process of directory searching is that you travel along a given route that, by definition, excludes other options the further you travel. When you get to the destination site the information might not be useful and you will have to move back one step or more to be able to view other pages. This takes a lot of time and it is easy to forget where you started from, or even what it was you were searching for. Indeed, there is so much choice in a directory that it is easy to be sidetracked and spend time on matters not directly related to what you really wanted to find. I hesitate to say 'waste' time because you will be practising your skills of directory searching and will be gaining awareness of just how much the Internet has to offer.

Storing site links in a 'favorites' folder

One way to avoid repetitive searches is to store favourite sites such as a specific information page or a directory service that you feel is easy to use. To store the link to that page in your 'favorites' folder do the following:

*   Step 1. Click on the menu word 'favorites'. The options 'add favorite' and 'organize favorites' will be displayed in a drop-down menu.
*   Step 2. Click on the first option. A window will appear with the fields 'name' and 'create in'.
*   Step 3. In the field 'name' you can type in a page title if the information auto-inserted is unclear. In the field 'create in' select whichever file you require. A non-selection will just add the link to the page beneath any files already present. In this way you are creating your own ready use directory.
*   Step 4. Click on the 'OK' button to save the Web page. You can also check the 'make available offline' box to be able to read the pages off line. This might not be necessary if you are on a network with open access to the Internet, but if you are paying for on-line time yourself it could allow you to download the site and browse it off line, thus saving money. This facility has an option to download links to three clicks from the main page.
*   Step 5. Click 'OK' to complete the action of saving a page link in 'favorites'.

Some browsers, such as Netscape Navigator, might have the term 'bookmarks' instead of 'favorites'.

So far a directory search has been used to browse through the sites selected and indexed by a given Internet company or organization. There are other general searching tools that will give an indication of content available on the Internet beyond that provided by a single company or organization. The next section deals with the rudiments of search engines.

Using a search engine

Search engines are online utilities that search thousands of Web documents quickly for a chosen word or phrase. It should be noted that no single search engine has the contents to every Web page on the Internet. This is why you might obtain different results from different search engines.

Three search engines will be discussed: a local search engine, which searches within a given site such as a directory; a meta-search engine, which searches several engines at once, and a subject-specific search engine.

Using a local search engine

A typical search engine appears as a field into which you type some text words of the topic you wish to search for, such as 'diabetes'. A phrase can also be typed in. You do not need to enter words like 'and', or 'the'. There are different types of engine, which will combine different combination of words 'and', 'or' and 'not'.

Controlled vocabulary and keyword searching

Librarians and other database producers have tried to solve problems of variety and ambiguity of language by creating *controlled vocabulary* for subject indexing in databases. They do this by selecting which of many possible terms (words or phrases) will be used for each concept in the database. Professional indexers review records as they are entered into the database and add controlled vocabulary terms to them so that all the items about the same topic will have the same subject heading or descriptor. The controlled vocabulary terms are entered into a special field in each record. In a database, controlled vocabulary terms are in the subject-headings field. Sometimes these are also called 'descriptors' or 'subjects'.

In a directory, the controlled vocabulary will be presented in terms of headings and subheadings and you will see these words underlined or highlighted as hypertext links. Another way to find controlled vocabulary terms is to use a thesaurus. A database thesaurus is similar to a language thesaurus. It lists synonyms and indicates relationships among terms. The database thesaurus often includes definitions for the chosen terms, explaining their meaning in the database. The thesaurus also lists synonyms that are not used in the database and directs the user from those to the chosen terms. Under a chosen term, the thesaurus lists other chosen terms that are more specific or more general. It may also list equally specific terms that are used for another facet of the chosen term. Using these terms in your search will help to ensure that you retrieve all the records relevant to your topic.

Most databases allow you to search by keyword. This type of search retrieves terms from both controlled vocabulary and free text fields. A keyword search usually retrieves more items than a controlled vocabulary search, but there is more chance that some of your results will not be relevant to your topic. This is because of ambiguity, which can come in with free text terms.

To help solve the problems of controlled vocabulary, database producers include searchable fields for free text terms in database records. Free text is 'uncontrolled vocabulary'. Concepts are expressed in free-text fields without reference to the database thesaurus. The usual free-text fields are title and abstract (if there are abstracts in your database). In some full-text databases, the entire text of the article is a free-text field. Authors of the articles, rather than indexers, are usually the ones who decide on the terms in free-text fields.

A keyword search is best when there is no descriptor or subject heading for your topic, the descriptor or subject heading is too general or too specific, you are searching for a new trend or concept, or the database you are searching does not have controlled vocabulary. Keyword searching can be a good way to begin your search. Find some relevant records in your results, then look at the descriptors or subject headings assigned to those records, and modify your search to include any of those terms that are relevant to your topic.

In many databases, you can choose between keyword searching and browse searching. Browse searching is sometimes called *exact searching* or *exact-match searching*. To search by this method you must enter your search terms in the order they appear in the field you are searching.

In browse searching, the computer matches letter for letter and space for space what you type in. The computer will return results for any records with fields beginning with the browse words you type in.

Truncation

The most commonly available form of truncation is right-hand truncation. This allows you to search for the first few letters of a word and retrieve any additional letters to the right. You may want to use right-hand truncation when you are looking for a word with different spellings, or different forms of a word, such as singular or plural forms and different endings. Using right-hand truncation, you will broaden your search and ensure that you retrieve all items containing a form of the word. For example, the truncation 'Politic*' will retrieve:

politic
politics
political
politically
politician
politicians

If you truncate a word too much you are likely to retrieve unwanted matches. For example, if you want all forms of the word culture, but type in cul*, you are likely to retrieve the following unwanted terms:

cult
cultivate
culinary
culminate
culottes
culprit

The best way to truncate this word is to type cultur*.

Two other forms of truncation are available in some databases.

One is wildcard truncation, in which you substitute a truncation symbol for one letter in a word. The letter could be within the word, as in 'wom#n', which may retrieve 'woman', 'women', 'womyn', 'womon', and so forth, or at the end, where it is usually used for plurals. Some databases allow you to specify the number of additional letters after the truncation by adding that many wildcard symbols to the word stem. The wildcard symbol is usually different from the right-hand truncation symbol.

The other form of truncation is left-hand truncation, which allows you to search for different prefixes on a word stem.

Truncation capabilities and symbols are different in different databases. Remember to check the online help information for the database you are searching to find out whether this feature is available and how to use it.

Boolean operators

Using the Boolean operators (AND, OR, NOT) to combine keywords in a database search allows you to narrow or expand your search. To build a complex search using two or more Boolean operators, you will need to learn the advanced technique of nesting.

- Use AND to narrow a search. *Both* terms must be present in any references you retrieve.
- Use OR to expand a search. Your search will retrieve records with *either* of the terms.
- Use NOT to exclude a term. Records with the first term will be retrieved, but any records with the second term will be eliminated.

Nesting involves the use of parentheses to insure that Boolean operations are performed in the sequence you intend. This technique allows you to build a complex search using two or more operators (AND, OR, NOT).

If you combine more than one different Boolean operator in a single search statement, you must use nesting for the search logic to work properly. If you are doing a search using only AND operators or only OR operators, you do not need to use nesting.

Here is a search statement using simple nesting: 'nursing AND (infants OR children)'. In this search the OR operation is nested and will be performed first. Then the AND operation will be performed. This search will retrieve items on nursing and infants and also on nursing and children.

Here is an example of a search statement using more complex nesting: '(smoking OR tobacco OR nicotine) AND (adolescents OR teenagers)'. The OR operations inside both sets of parentheses will be performed first, and then the resulting sets will be combined using the AND operator. Nesting synonyms in this way can broaden your search.

Here is an example of a search statement in which the logic is not properly stated: smoking OR tobacco AND adolescents OR teenagers. This search will perform the OR and AND operations in the sequence that they are typed. It will retrieve items on smoking, articles on tobacco and adolescents, and articles on teenagers. The logic can be corrected by nesting the two OR statements: '(smoking OR tobacco) AND (adolescents OR teenagers)'.

Altering the search engine parameters

Somewhere near the search engine field will be a button to click on with the word GO or SEARCH or some other similar term. You can find search engines located on most directory services. Some will be specific to the directory. A typical example is to be found on the Yahoo! Web page, http://uk.yahoo.com. The directory displays a simple search engine into which you type a search term. If you want to refine your search you can get some tips and set some search parameters by clicking on 'advanced search'. Most search engines provide additional guidance help on searching. In this case the extra options are:

- to search with an intelligent default
- to search an exact phrase match
- to search for matches on all words (and)
- to search for matches on any word (or).

A second parameter is to select either Yahoo! categories or Web sites. A third parameter is to find listings added during the past number of years, months, weeks or days. The fourth parameter offered is to display the number of matches per page in increments from 10 to 100. It is quicker to display as many as possible so as not to have to keep clicking on the 'next page' icon to read the next 10 or so hits. It is important to understand that to refine your search and focus on relevant information you must select your search terms and set the search engine parameters to filter out irrelevant information.

Setting search engine parameters.

There might be additional tips on how to achieve this by clicking a button near the search engine. The 'additional tips' for a Yahoo! search engine are:

Required and prohibited search words.
Attaching an operator: Plus [+] or minus [–] will either require or prohibit words from appearing in the search results.
+ Attached to a word requires that the word be found in all of the search results.
compare police versus police +sting

– Attached to a word requires that the word not be found in any of the search results.
compare python versus python -monty

For example, 'dog -hound' produced results for 241 Web pages whereas 'dog +hound' produced 16 categories, 108 sites and 35,700 Web pages. The Yahoo! example continues:

Document selection restrictions.
Attaching one of the following operators to the front of a search word will restrict the search to . . . certain document sections.

t: will restrict searches to document titles only.
compare joe boxer versus t:joe boxer

u: will restrict searches to document URLs only
compare intel versus u:intel

For example t:dog+hound produced 16 categories, 89 sites and one Web page with the words 'dog' and 'hound' in the title. U:dog+hound produced 0 categories, five sites and only one Web page with the terms in the URL.

Phrase matching (" ")
Putting words in quote marks will find only results that match words in that exact sequence.
compare great barrier reef versus "great barrier reef"

An example is 'north sea', producing 0 categories and 200 sites, and "north sea", which produced 0 categories and 26 sites.

> Wildcard matching
> Attaching a * to the right-hand side of a word will return left side partial matches.
> *compare* cap and cap*

The former returned 23 categories and 1,324 sites. The latter returned 353 categories and 19,254 sites.

> Combining the syntax
> You may combine any of the query syntax as long as the syntax is combined in the proper order. The proper order for using the is . . . +, −, t:, u:, "" and lastly *.

Overall, the principle should be the same with different search engines found on Web pages. If in doubt check out the specific advice given with each search engine that you use.

Using a search engine – an example

Using the engine on the Yahoo! page mentioned above, the search term "diabetes diagnosis" using the parameters of search method: 'exact phrase', new listings: 'over the last 6 months' and search area 'Yahoo! Categories' produced only one hit:

> Yahoo! Site Matches (1 – 1 of 1)
> Health > Diseases and Conditions > Diabetes
> Jamila Diabetes & Endocrine Center 06/15/2000 discusses diagnosis, treatment, and complications of diabetes, as well as thyroid and other endocrine disorders. Offers weekly case studies for physicians.

Your search words will often be highlighted in the result. The next example shows how altering the parameter alters the number of hits returned. First the search engine was used on the Yahoo! page and the search terms 'Elderly care' were typed into the field. The 'all of Yahoo!' selection was made and the search returned no categories, 263 sites and 237,000 Web pages. Altering the selection to 'UK only' reduced the number of sites located to 22.

It will be apparent to you by now that there is a need to be able to refine your search so as to remove from your view all of the irrelevant material. The key to this is to be able to select relevant search words and set appropriate search parameters. Having said this, a general directory search can be a good starting place to scan through the range of material available on a given topic.

Metasearches – using several search engines at once

A metasearch uses more than one search engine at a time. If one search engine looks at the indexed site of only one Internet organization then it would be more efficient to use several engines at once. This is possible, and sites where such search facilities are available include:

- Coppernic.com, at http://www.coppernic.com, advertises itself as a 'Powerful and easy to use search tool [that] will consult the best Internet search engines for you and bring back relevant, sorted and filtered results.' You can download a free search program from that Web site.
- Mamma.com, at http://www.mamma.com, markets itself as the 'mother of all search engines'.
- Google.com is another such metasearch engine that produces results by relevance to your enquiry. The information found at http://www.google.com/why_use.html gives more details about the benefits of this search engine.

Each metasearch engine has slight variations about how it is configured. For example the 'advanced search' on Google.com has a variety of additional search features:

- restrict your search to pages within a given Web site;
- exclude pages from a particular Web site;
- restrict your search to pages only in a given language;
- find all the pages that link to a given Web page;
- find pages that are related to a given Web page.

The example of a Dogpile metasearch (www.dogpile.com) is shown next. The search term 'decision making theory' was required. The result produced the following:

Search engine: Looksmart found 5 results.
</>http://www.looksmart.com//> The query string sent was +decision +making +theory
Search engine: GoTo.com found 10 or more results.
</>http://www.goto.com/>
Search engine: FindWhat.com found 0 results.
</>http:www.findwhat.com//> The query string sent was decision making theory.
Search engine: Direct Hit found 10 or more results. </>www.directhit.com/>
The query string sent was +decision+making+theory.
Search engine: Google found 258,000 results. </>http://click.go2net.com/>
The query string sent was decision making theory.
Search engine: Sprinks from About found 353 results.
</>http://search.sprinks.about.com/index./>The query string sent was +decision +making +theory.
Search engine: Infoseek found 0 results </>http://infoseek.go.com/> The query string sent was decision making theory.
Search engine: Lycos found 10 or more results.
</>http://www.lycos.com//> The query string sent was +decision +making +theory.
Search engine: Dogpile Open Directory found 1 result.
</>http://opendir.dogpile.com//> The query string sent was decision making theory.
Search engine: RealNames found 10 or more results.
</>http://navigation.realnames.com//>The query string sent was decision making theory.
Search engine: AltaVista found 9750 results.
</>http://www.altavista.com//> The query string sent was +decision +making +theory.
Search engine: Yahoo found 3 results. </>http://www.yahoo.com//> The query string sent was +decision +making +theory.

It also generated a specific directory asking: 'are you looking for?'

Decision making.
Location theory.
Career decision-making theories.
Edward Tufte,
Descriptive theories of decision making,
RWS publications,
Theorie decision,
Egan theory of career decision-making.

You might have gathered by now that you need to explore your choice of search engines and the parameters of each if they are to work efficiently for you.

Using a subject-specific search engine

This is a search engine that searches only within a given focus. It is subject specific. First, you need to find a directory of subject-specific search engines. Try the site http://www.beaucoup.com. Beaucoup.com contains some 2,500 search engines under a range of categories. Select the category and locate from the subsequent directory a search engine dealing with your topic area. It also includes a metasearcher that uses several search engines at once.

Plain language searches

There are search engines that allow you to type in a plain language (free text) enquiry. They will find a range of answers near to your submission. Some of these engines might automatically match your search words to MeSH headings.

MeSH is the National Library of Medicine's controlled vocabulary thesaurus. Thesauri are carefully constructed sets of terms often connected by 'broader-than', 'narrower-than', and 'related' links. These links show the relationship between related terms and provide a hierarchical structure that permits searching at various levels of specificity from narrower to broader. Thesauri are also known as 'classification structures', 'controlled vocabularies', and 'ordering systems'.

MeSH consists of a set of terms or subject headings that are arranged in both an alphabetic and a hierarchical structure. At the most general level of the hierarchical structure are very broad headings such as 'Anatomy', 'Mental Disorders', and 'Enzymes, Coenzymes, and Enzyme Inhibitors'. At more narrow levels are found more specific headings such as 'Ankle', 'Conduct Disorder', and 'Calcineurin'. There are more than 19,000 main headings in MeSH. In addition to these headings, there are 103,500 headings called Supplementary Concept Records (formerly Supplementary Chemical Records) within a separate chemical thesaurus. There are also thousands of cross-references that assist in finding the most appropriate MeSH Heading, for example, Vitamin C see Ascorbic Acid.
(Source: http://www.nlm.nih.gov/pubs/factsheets/mesh.html.)

Once the plain text metasearcher has displayed results (and some of these offer further opportunities to refine the search) you are in a position to explore a relevant-looking site or initiate a further search within the selections offered.

A good example of this type of search engine is 'Ask Jeeves' at http://www.ask.co.uk. The results for a plain text enquiry of 'find me: Nursing databases' included points where further enquiry could be initiated by clicking on the 'ask' button; some resources found on OnHealth.com; some resources based on answers to questions asked by others; and a directory of related search terms.

Points where a further enquiry could be initiated.
ASK Where can I ask a doctor about disease areas?
ASK Where can I find resources from Britannica.com on nurse?
ASK What are the top graduate programs in nursing according to U.S News & World Report?
ASK What should I know to choose the physician that's right for me?

OnHealth.com has the following relevant information:
Drug Database
One-stop searching in the most comprehensive medical conditions and pharmacy databases online, interactive anatomy charts and food pyramids, and assessment tests.
Angelica Root
One-stop searching in the most comprehensive medical conditions and pharmacy databases online, interactive anatomy charts and food pyramids, and assessment tests.
Job Opportunities at OnHealth Network Company
Company information, including how to contact us; advertising opportunities; investor relations and job postings.

People with similar questions have found these sites relevant:
Ask The Nurses
Ask the Nurses, Medical Questions, Telemedicine, Ask The Doctor, Fibromyalgia, CFIDS, Medical Library, Myalgic Encephalomyelitis, Medical Chat, Medical Links, Medical News
Search the Licensed Practical Nurse Database

For a more specific search, use the first name or initial. For example, to search for Jane Smith, enter SMITH J or SMITH JANE. Do not use commas or periods.
OR
Search by
Nursing Databases, Search engines
nursing search engines and databases @ MedNets
Medical/health/fitness experts

(contd)

Medicine Ask An Orthopedist Ask An STD Specialist Ask a Mayo Clinic Physician Ask an Oral Maxillofacial Surgeon Ask the Optometrist Ask the Pharma-
cist Ask a Fertility and
ENW: Emergency Nursing World! (http://ENW.org)
Emergency Nursing World!

You may also wish to try these related searches:
Nurses Database
Databases For Nursing Education
Nursing Informatics Terminology Database
Nursing Database Nurse CINHAL
Nurses Education Italy
Nursing Times
Ask Nurse
Emergency Nurses
Nurse Chat

The advantage of these search engines is that they can help you to
refine your search and they can also generate academic and professional links. The next stage is to refine the focus of the search. This
necessarily means deselecting a huge amount of information and
determining to work in just one part of the whole array of possible
information. In the preceding example some of the links led to
searchable clinical databases and part or full-text journal articles.

Database searching: tools to locate professional information

The quickest way to find professional subject-specific databases is to
link through 'professional' sites (political and academic). These can
be found through directory and general metasearches, which generate specific URLs. Another approach is to search through political,
global organization and academic sites – use the list at the end of this
chapter to help to get you started. Most of these 'professional' sites
will offer links to a range of similar discipline-based areas of information. The World Health Organization (http://www.who.int/) for
example, has links to information sources on its home page including
documents, bulletins, reports and statistical information and a
further link to databases on the Web. If you follow that link you will
find several free and high-quality databases.

Examples of such professional and academic sites are:

Medical

- The National Library of Medicine (http://www.nlm.nih.gov/).
- Medic8.com – a UK Medical portal (http://www.medic8.com/MedicalDatabases.htm).

Nursing

- NMAP is a Nursing Midwifery and Allied Health professions gateway to internet resources. It is found at http://nmap.ac.uk It is aimed at students, researchers, academics and practitioners to enable users to get quick and efficient access to reliable health information. It is a component of ONMI (Organising Medical Networked Information) and is based in Nottingham University. ONMI and NMAP form part of BIOME, the health and life science hub of the national Resource Discovery Network (RDN). The RDN http://www.rdn.ac.uk provides a range of subject based internet services.

Health generally

- The Internet Sleuth Health Databases Collection (http://www.isleuth.com/heal.html). This is a page of searchable databases with a US emphasis.
- The NHS Centre for Reviews and Dissemination found on the University of York Web site (http://www.york.ac.uk/) has links to the following databases:
  - Database of Abstracts of Reviews of Effectiveness (DARE) (http://agatha.york.ac.uk/darehp.htm). This is a database of high-quality systematic research reviews of the effectiveness of health care interventions.
  - NHS Economic Evaluation Database (NHS EED) (http://agatha.york.ac.uk/nhsdhp.htm). The NHS Economic Evaluation Database is a database of structured abstracts of economic evaluations of health care interventions.
  - Health Technology Assessment database (HTA) (http://agatha.york.ac.uk/htahp.htm). The HTA database contains abstracts produced by INAHTA and other health care technology agencies.

- – This Web site also has some online articles about undertaking searches using MEDLINE and CINAHL. These are located at http://www.york.ac.uk/inst/crd/search.htm under the heading 'Search Strategies to Identify Reviews and Meta-analyses in MEDLINE and CINAHL' and give detailed guidance about conducting a metasearch using the two databases.
- The Department of Health home page on the UK government Web site (http://www.open.gov.uk) has links to all the NHS departments and publicly funded initiatives to develop clinical practice. It is found at http://www.doh.gov.uk/.

Social science

- The Social Science Information Gateway (SOSIG) http://sosig.ac.uk/. This allows you to set up a (free) personal registration page, which has facilities to link you to others having similar interests.

The Social Science Information Gateway (SOSIG) aims to provide a trusted source of selected, high quality Internet information for researchers and practitioners in the social sciences, business and law. It is part of the UK Resource Discovery Network.

. . . The SOSIG Internet Catalogue is an online database of high quality Internet resources. It offers users the chance to read descriptions of resources available over the Internet and to access those resources directly. The Catalogue points to thousands of resources, and each one has been selected and described by a librarian or academic. The catalogue is browsable or searchable by subject area.

. . . This is a database of over 50,000 Social Science Web pages. Whereas the resources found in the SOSIG Internet Catalogue have been selected by subject experts, those in the Social Science Search Engine have been collected by software called a 'harvester' (similar mechanisms may be referred to as 'robots' or 'Web crawlers'). All the pages collected stem from the main Internet catalogue this provides the equivalent of a social science search engine.
(source: http://wwww.Sosig.ac.uk/)

Academia generally

- There is an academic directory search facility at http://acdc.hensa.ac.uk/index.shtml.
- A useful interactive university finder for the British Isles can be found on the University of Wolverhampton Web site at http://www.scit.wlv.ac.uk/ukinfo/uk.map.html.

Once a database has been found you will usually recognize a search engine for that database and a means of refining the search. Some sites have facilities to e-mail the results of the search to you or print off material. Some will even provide full text articles for free whilst others will require a payment. The instructions will be clear on the screen.

Parameters of a database.

When working within databases it is good to think about the specific ways of limiting the search. A good technique for refining or focusing a database search is to limit your search to a specific field. Remember, a field is an individual element of information in a record. Here are some examples of fields:

- title
- author
- subject
- journal or source
- publication year
- language
- abstract.

You may want to do a field-specific search when you are looking for:

- articles in a particular journal
- items published in a particular year or years
- publications written by a particular person.

Sometimes the author field is controlled, meaning that the database has a standard way of entering authors' names, and all authors' names are in the same format. Sometimes the author field is free text, meaning that the names can be in different formats. In either case, the names may or may not appear as they do in the publication being indexed. For this reason it may be necessary, or a good idea, to use truncation in searching for an author's name. Remember to check out the help page for each database to find out how to do a field-specific search in it.

Practice

There is no substitute for practice to develop your searching skills. Begin by selecting a search term of personal interest and try using it with different types of searches to see what type of results you retrieve. Think carefully about the words you use to conceptualize this topic. Then start with a general search using a commercial directory such as Yahoo! or Microsoft Network. Navigate your way through the directory until you get near to the information sought.

Next use the search engine on the commercial directory to see the types of results that are retrieved. Try altering the parameters of the search engine and of the search words themselves to refine (focus) the enquiry.

Next try searching several directories at once using a metasearch engine such as Dog Pile. Again, navigate your way through a selected directory link from the results to see what information you can find related to your topic focus.

Next use a plain text metasearch engine such as 'Ask Jeeves', www.ask.co.uk. Type in plain English what it is you are looking for and navigate your way down through the results selecting something that looks relevant to your enquiry.

The above search will probably produce several URLs – go directly to an information location using one of those links.

Find a professional database either in the academic or political domain. Navigate your way within a database (this might be a full-text journal site where you can view every article in issues stretching back a number of years). Try one of the examples mentioned in the text if the plain text search engine did not produce any professional database URLs.

Having completed those searches try sketching out a conceptual map of the information domain considered and the nature of information seen on screen. It might be helpful to take a sheet of paper and lay out professional, commercial, personal interest Web sites, and academic Web sites. There will be further subdivisions within each section, for example professional practice, research and policy headings. It is also worth storing selected sites in your 'favorites' folder and perhaps keeping a notebook record too.

Information-finding aids: search engines

Listed below are some search engines available on the Web. This is in no way intended to be a comprehensive list.

http://www.infoseek.com

http://www.excite.com

http://www.lycos.com

http://www.yahoo.com

http://www.mckinley.com

http://index.opentext.net

http://nln.com

http://altavista.digital.com

http://www.hotbot.com

http://www.webcrawler.com

Web guides/Web directories

Web guides are guides to information available on the Web, sorted by topic. Each guide contains only those pages entered into it by its compiler, so they are not comprehensive. Some contain a vast variety of topics whereas others include topics related to a specific field, such as education or music, for example. You can usually browse or search the guides. A few of the available Web guides are:

http://a2z.lycos.com

http://www.albert2.com

http://point.lycos.con

http://www.yahoo.com

Yellow Pages

These are directory-based listings of Internet sites (primarily Web pages) and their URLs by categories (in alphabetical order), similar to the *Yellow Pages* directories. These books can be found at computer stores and at most bookstores. If you type the search term 'International yellow pages' into the search engine on http://www.msn.com/ you will have access to a directory of at least 60 *Yellow Pages* results.

Chapter 7
Using e-mail for networking

Introduction

E-mail is simply a way to send messages to another person using a computer or hand-held device. The latest technology means that you do not even have to have a cable link to the telephone system. Most computers have a modem, which is connected by a wire to your telephone line, and a message sent is routed via a line to another computer. There are several e-mail devices now, including e-mail landline telephones, e-mail mobile telephones, and digital communications (through your TV). This chapter deals with the use of e-mail with a computer connected to a network through a physical cable link. It is a portable means of communication in that wherever you are in the world all you have to do is dial the ISP and then, assuming you can connect to it, you will be able to retrieve your mail. It can also provide you with a permanent address where you can be contacted regardless of where you are in the world.

There are several e-mail programs available and most of them are free. If you bought a computer it might well have come preloaded with software such as Microsoft Outlook Express. Free e-mail accounts also come with Internet service providers such as Freeserve. E-mail accounts are also available via the Web, with Hotmail and Yahoo! being two examples.

The principles of using e-mail are essentially the same whichever service provider you use. You can create and send mail, you can receive and read mail, you can stop unwanted mail and you can send documents as attachments to the e-mail.

The e-mail can include pictures and sounds as well as documents – for example a word-processed file or a Web page html file. Your messages can have hyperlinks too, so that the reader can, at the click of the mouse, open up a Web address that you have sent to them.

When reading mail you can reply straight away, compose a new message or just store the message in a folder that you have created.

The e-mail address

In the same way that a house has a postal address so with an e-mail account you have an e-mail address. This consists of the user ID and the domain name of the ISP. When written it looks like this:

username@company.co.uk

You will see many examples of these on posters and increasingly on letterheads and in publications. The username does not have to have your actual name, mine for example is the name of my Web service – Prepare. My full address is prepare@globalnet.co.uk.

This means that my username is prepare, the ISP is Globalnet and Globalnet's domain name is Globalnet.co.uk (to pronounce this you would say 'prepare at Globalnet dot co dot uk'). It is essential to type e-mail addresses accurately and the dots between words (called periods) are parts of the address. If you accidentally type in a space this will be read as a different address and probably will not be able to find the electronic destination.

There are a couple of easy ways to find e-mail addresses. One is to look at an e-mail that has been sent to you and look at the 'from' line in the header of the letter. If you right click on this you will usually be given the option from a pop-up menu to save it in your address book. Next you could check through an e-mail directory of the company or organization where the addressee is based. Many companies and organizations with Web pages have listings of contacts within their organization. These often give you telephone numbers and e-mail addresses. You could also try out one of the many sites on the Internet that provide 'search for people' search facilities. These are listed in the resources section at the end of this chapter, and the chapter on using the Internet browser will guide you through how to find them.

Setting up an e-mail account

To set up an e-mail account you will need to choose an ISP. There are many offering free e-mail, and software is available from ISP Web Sites or on free CDRoms.

Growing familiar with the e-mail window

To open the e-mail application click on the icon on your desktop or find it on the task bar along the bottom of the screen or in the 'start' menu. This section refers to Microsoft Outlook Express which has a familiar window with a title bar, a menu bar and a toolbar with buttons. If you launch the application you can work through the text and identify specific functions on screen.

The appearance of the window can be altered to suit your preferences by clicking on the 'view' menu and selecting 'layout' from the menu. A series of check boxes allow you a number of options before clicking on 'apply' to effect the changes. If you do not like the new layout just go back into the menu and alter the selections. You can also size the window, as shown previously, by clicking and dragging the frame border. To move the window, click and drag the title bar and 'drop' it where you want it.

You will notice that on the left-hand side of the window there is a pane showing a list of files. If one of these is selected its contents will appear in the right-hand pane.

The local folders will have 'inbox', 'sent items', 'deleted items', 'drafts' and any other folders you might have created. If you click on inbox so that it is highlighted (has a blue bar over it) the contents of the inbox will appear in the right-hand pane. Highlighting an item in the right-hand pane will show its contents in the lower right pane, which is called the *preview pane*. Once again, you can set the position of the preview pane as being at the side of or underneath the contents pane. If you double click on the mail in the top right pane the letter will be shown in a new window. An up and down arrow on the toolbar will allow you to switch between all messages in your inbox. The same applies if you are checking through messages stored in a folder.

The other folder shown in this view is the newsgroup list. This will be discussed later.

To compose and send an e-mail message

It is easy to do this. You start by clicking on the 'new mail' button on the toolbar. The same action can also be achieved by clicking on the menu 'file' and selecting from the drop down menu 'compose new mail'. A window will appear that has 'address' and 'message' title bars and a large space for the main body of the message.

First, type in the address of the person to whom you are sending your mail. Click the mouse pointer in the field so that the cursor is seen in it and then type the address. Remember that the address must be correct: the position of the dots must be correct and do not use spaces unless included in the address otherwise the e-mail system will return the message as undeliverable – 'addressee unknown'.

The 'to' field is the primary recipient and the 'cc' field is for 'carbon copies' to be sent to other people. You can type more than one name in these fields. To remember addresses you can set up an address book, which is created through clicking on the 'tools' menu and selecting 'address book'. That opens a window in which you can create a new address by following the instructions in the window. You can move between fields to type in details either by clicking the mouse on the next field or by pressing the 'tab' key on the keyboard. This key is on the left-hand side of the keyboard and has two arrows pointing in opposite directions. Once the address book has been created and the window has been closed you can call up addresses by clicking on the book icon next to the word 'to' at the address bar. This will open your address book and you can click on the address required, click the button so that the address moves into the message recipient's window and then click 'OK' to complete the action and close the address book window. The addressee will appear in the 'to' or 'cc' field, depending on which address book icon was clicked.

If you type two or more e-mail names in the 'to' and/or 'cc' boxes they must be separated by a comma or semicolon.

In the 'subject' box, type a message title. If you don't when you send the letter a message screen will appear asking if you want to send it without a title. You should always include a title.

The main text of your message is typed in the body of the window and then, when completed, all you do is click on the 'send' icon on the new message toolbar. If at that stage you are working offline (on a home PC for example) a message screen will appear asking if you want to back online now. If you click 'OK', the ISP will be dialled and, once a connection is established, the message will be sent.

When you click the icon 'send' or the menu 'file'/'send' the ISP will be dialled and a window will list the actions taking place, such as 'sending two messages' and 'retrieving mail from server'. It is worth checking the 'hang up when completed' box by clicking it with the mouse so that you do not incur unnecessary telephone online charges. When it is selected a small tick will be displayed in the box.

Working online and offline

You can reduce your telephone bill by working offline as much as possible. When you click on the e-mail icon to launch the application then a window will appear asking if you want to go online. This can be set up to dial up the connection automatically once you click the e-mail icon. The application opens and any new mail is transferred from the server to your computer. You can then, if you have selected 'inbox' in the folders pane, view a list of new mail. You do not have to be online to read it, so you can either set your connection up to hang up on completion of sending and receiving mail or click on the 'work offline' icon. If, after a short while, you want to send a new message all you have to do is click on the 'work online' icon and you will be connected up again.

If you work offline for a given amount of time the connection will be automatically terminated. To adjust this setting, click on the menu 'tools'/'options'. A tabbed page will appear from which you need to select the 'connections' tab. There will be a graphic entitled 'dial up' and you need to check (click on) the small white field so that an x appears relating to the statement 'hang up after sending and receiving'.

If you are composing a message offline, your message will be saved in the outbox. It will be sent automatically when you go back online. When closing down your system a message screen might appear and remind you that you have unsent messages and ask if they should be sent now. Click 'OK' if you want this.

Draft messages

You might be drafting a message and want to work on it later on. To save a draft click the 'file' menu and then click 'save'. You can also click 'save as' to save a mail message in your file system in mail (eml), text (.txt), or HTML (htm) format. The draft will be accessible through the 'drafts' folder of your 'folders' window in the left-hand pane. The simplest way to become familiar with these actions is to practise. Send messages to friends and get them to reply.

Attaching items to a message

It can be very useful to insert a document file in a message, for example to allow someone to read a report, minutes of a meeting or some other information too lengthy to type into the body of an e-mail. To insert a file in a message click anywhere in the message window.

In the 'insert' menu, click 'file attachment'. A window will appear similar to that in the word processor when you click 'file'/'open'. Select the location and then the file within that location. When it has been found, select it and click 'attach', and then find the file you want to attach. The file will now be listed in the 'attach' box in the message header. You can complete the same action by clicking on the attach icon, which looks like a paper clip. You can also add a text (*.txt) file into the body of your mail message by clicking the 'insert' menu and then clicking 'text' from 'file'. You select the file required so that it appears in the file name field and then click 'OK'. The text will then appear in the body of the message.

To insert a picture in a message

Click where you want the image to appear in the message. In the 'insert' menu, click 'picture', and then click 'browse' to find the image file. A window will appear and you can click the 'browse' button to locate the image file if you are not sure what to type in the image source field. Enter layout and spacing information for the image file as required and click 'OK'. The image will appear in the text of your document.

To insert a hyperlink or HTML page in a message.

In the message window, click where you want to add the hyperlink or Web-page text. To add a hyperlink, click the 'insert' menu, and then click 'hyperlink'. Select the file type, and then type the location or address of the link. To add an HTML page, click the 'insert' menu, and then click 'text from file'. Change the 'files of type' box to 'HTML files' and then find the file you want to add.

If you cannot select the hyperlink menu command, make sure HTML formatting is turned on by clicking the 'format' menu in the message window and then clicking rich text (HTML). A black dot appears by the command when it is selected.

Finding e-mail addresses

If you want to search an e-mail directory many of the commercial search engines such as Yahoo!, Netscape and Lycos have finding aids.

Privacy and e-mail

It is probably fair to say that privacy cannot be guaranteed. So it is necessary to take some steps to protect your files and e-mail from being read by someone else. One simple barrier is password protection but it is not infallible. To find how to set it up (using Windows 98) click 'start'/'settings'/'control panel' and when it opens select the icon 'users' and the dialogue box will lead you through a series of steps that will allow you to create a password and parameters of your personal desktop screen. Having set up the system to allow access by more than one user you can change the password if you wish by clicking on the 'change password' icon in the control panel.

Sending secure messages

As more people send confidential information by e-mail, it is increasingly important to be sure that documents sent in e-mail are not forged and to be certain that messages you send cannot be intercepted and read by anyone other than your intended recipient. To help maintain privacy you will need to get a 'digital ID'. This allows you to prove your identity in electronic transactions in a way similar to showing your cash guarantee card when you cash a check. You can also use your digital ID to encrypt messages, keeping them private.

How do digital IDs work?

A digital ID is composed of a 'public key', a 'private key', and a 'digital signature'. When you digitally sign your messages you are adding your digital signature and public key to the message. The combination of a digital signature and public key is called a 'certificate'.

Recipients can use your digital signature to verify your identity and use your public key to send you encrypted mail that only you can read by using your private key. In order to send encrypted messages, your address book must contain digital IDs for the recipients. You use their public key to encrypt the messages. When recipients get encrypted messages, their private key is used to decrypt the message for reading.

Before you can start sending digitally signed messages you must obtain a digital ID and set up your mail account to use it. If you are sending encrypted messages, your address book must contain a digital ID for each recipient.

Where do you get digital IDs?

Digital IDs are issued by independent certification authorities. When you apply for a digital ID at a certification authority's Web site, they verify your identity before issuing an ID. There are different classes of digital IDs, each certifying a different level of trustworthiness. The Web sites allow you to verify the validity of a digitally signed message. More information on this can be found at the help file at the certification authority's Web site. There is a charge for a digital ID.

There are three ways to obtain someone else's digital ID. You can ask them to send you digitally signed mail, or you can search the digital ID database on a certification authority's Web site. You can also search Internet directory services that list digital IDs along with other properties. One digital ID verification www site is: http:// digitalid.verisign.com/.

Networking

Networking is often seen as a means of collaborating with others for mutual benefit. Whilst it conjures up images of 'the old school tie' and 'who you know', that is not the type of network under discussion here. A professional network is, in its simplest form, a discussion forum for sharing ideas and information. You might never meet the people in the network but you can develop worldwide links related to your area of interest. The benefits of joining a networked community include information sharing, keeping in touch with current debates in your field, getting to ask questions about clinical practice and receiving advice.

Where are networks to be found?

There are two main sources that enable you to find networks. One is via your e-mail software and the second is by the Internet. The e-mail lists will be discussed first and then a professional network found on the Web. Both of these use e-mail as the means of communication. A third way of finding networks is also by the Internet and involves online discussions.

There are two e-mail-based discussion forums that are useful to sharing professional knowledge. One is the Mailbase list and the second newsgroups. The newsgroups are part of commercial ISP services and apart from professional interest groups are more akin to hobby groups and some have offensive and pornographic content.

Mailbase

Mailbase is a service that runs a series of e-mail-based discussion lists for UK academics and support staff. The discussion list is a group of people who share a common interest, such as evidence-based medicine, and join a list and use e-mail to talk to one another. Belonging to a list is the same as sitting in on a discussion. You can chose to join in or just observe. You might want to do this at first to get a feel for the way the list works. This is called *lurking*.

The list works by sending a message to the Mailbase computer. This might be to a group called 'evidence-based health' or 'evidence-based medicine' for example. Any member of the group can initiate a discussion or ask for information about some specific topic. All members receive that message by e-mail and can then send back replies and so the conversation between those who participate develops. The Mailbase WWW sites can be found at http://www.liszt.com and http://www.mailbase.ac.uk.

How to subscribe

To join a list (subscribe) point your Internet browser to a site such as http://www.jiscmail.ac.uk and search for the relevant list by keyword or subject. You join by sending a command in the body of an e-mail message to the Mailbase computer. The instructions will be on the Web site. You send a message to mailbase@mailbase.ac.uk. Type in the body of the message, join list name, first name, and last name. For example 'join evidence-based medicine jack smith'. Then click 'send' on your e-mail button bar.

How to post a message to a list

If you want to send a message to all the members of the group then send an e-mail message to: listname@mailbase.ac.uk where listname is the name of the list subscribed to. You automatically receive e-mails posted to the list group. However, if you are going away and do not want to come home to have to wade through scores of e-mails then you can suspend reception of mail from the group. This temporarily halts e-mail from the list. Send a message to jiscmail@jiscmail.ac.uk and type in the body of the e-mail

    suspend mail listname

(Type the name of your list instead of 'listname'.) When you want to start receiving e-mail again send this message to ac.uk:

    resume-mail listname

(where listname is the name of your list). If you belong to several lists then you can suspend all mail by sending the following message to jiscmail@ jiscmail.ac.uk:

    suspend mail ALL

To start receiving mail again from all of your lists then send the message:

    resume-mail ALL

If you have forgotten the Mailbase lists to which you are subscribed send an e-mail to jiscmail@ jiscmail.ac.uk and type in the body of the message:

    list me

To get the names and addresses of all other list members send an
e-mail message to jiscmail@ jiscmail.ac.uk with the following typed
in the body of the message:

> review list name

(where list name is the name of your list). You can read old messages
on the list by visiting the Web page at
http://www.mailbase.ac.uk/lists/list name/ (where list name is the
name of the list you wish to view).

To send a message to the list is quite simple. All you do is address
your e-mail to

> list name@jiscmail.ac.uk

(where list name is the name of particular list) and then type your
message in the body of the e-mail and click 'send'.

Once you are a member of a list there are certain guidelines
about acceptable use and list 'etiquette'. These are found on the Web
site, as is further information about the service and how to ask for
help if you have a problem such as leaving a list or sending a
message.

Nurse-decision archives – August 1999 (By Subject)
Previous month | Next month | Other months | Search | List Homepage
21 Messages sorted by: [author] [date] [thread]
Starting: Tue 03 Aug 1999 – 12:05:29 BST
Ending: Tue 31 Aug 1999 – 23:32:51 BST
(Fwd) A starting point . . . clinical questions
name (Tue 10 Aug 1999 – 16:34:01 BST)
A starting point . . . clinical questions
 name (Tue 10 Aug 1999 – 15:13:35 BST)
critically appraised topic
name (Tue 31 Aug 1999 – 15:07:25 BST)
eb on call and clinical questions
name (Mon 09 Aug 1999 – 12:28:28 BST)
name (Mon 09 Aug 1999 – 09:47:46 BST)
evidence base on call
name (Thu 05 Aug 1999 – 01:09:42 BST)
evidence based 'on call'
(Wed 04 Aug 1999 – 01:02:55 BST)

(contd)

evidence based on call (fwd)
name (Thu 05 Aug 1999 – 09:53:48 BST)
name (Thu 05 Aug 1999 – 09:48:47 BST)
name (Wed 04 Aug 1999 – 16:58:51 BST)
name (Wed 04 Aug 1999 – 15:27:47 BST)
evidence-based On-call
name (Tue 03 Aug 1999 – 12:05:25 BST)
important chance to influence health info.
name (Thu 12 Aug 1999 – 11:49:38 BST)
Next year's symposium on nurse decision-making.
name (Tue 31 Aug 1999 – 09:49:13 BST)
Notification of Conference – Progress 2000
name (Thu 26 Aug 1999 – 10:52:06 BST)
PEG feeding CAT posted on mailbase website – comments please.
name (Tue 31 Aug 1999 – 11:58:16 BST)
service users & multidisciplinary decisions
name (Thu 26 Aug 1999 – 14:36:10 BST)
Specialists in care of older people
name (Fri 06 Aug 1999 – 15:29:01 BST)
study
name (Sun 01 Aug 1999 – 14:34:01 BST)
UNSUBSCRIBE
name (Tue 31 Aug 1999 – 23:30:23 BST)
Last message date: Tue 31 Aug 1999 – 23:32:51 BST
Archived on: Thu 02 Sep 1999 – 01:44:06 BST
21 Messages sorted by: [author] [date] [thread]
Previous month | Next month | Other months | Search | List Homepage
Archive generated by hypermail 2a23: Thu 02 Sep 1999 – 01:44:06 BST
Figure 7.1 Example archive of a list discussion from the Mailbase Web site (names removed for privacy)

You can get journals and other sites automatically to send you e-mails about the contents of the latest issue or current job vacancies. For Jobs try www.jobs.ac.uk, and for journals try http://www.biomednet.com/ or http://www.elsevier.nl/ and you will find that you can select a number of journals from a given list and set up a preferences page to notify you of the contents at each issue date.

Newsgroups

A newsgroup is a collection of messages posted by individuals to a news server, a computer that can host thousands of newsgroups. You can find newsgroups on practically any subject. Although some newsgroups are moderated, most are not. Moderated newsgroups are 'owned' by someone who reviews the postings, can answer questions, delete inappropriate messages, and so forth. Anyone can post messages to a newsgroup. Newsgroups do not require any kind of membership or joining fees.

To use newsgroups in Outlook Express, your Internet service provider must offer links to one or more news servers. After you set up an account in Outlook Express for each server you want, you can read and post messages in any of the newsgroups stored on that news server.

When you find a newsgroup you like, you can 'subscribe' to it so that it is displayed in your Outlook Express Folders list. Subscribing provides easy access to your favourite newsgroups, eliminating the need to scroll through the long list on the server each time you want to visit a favourite newsgroup.

Newsgroups can contain thousands of messages, which can be time consuming to sort through. Outlook Express has a variety of features that make it easier to find the information you want in newsgroups. The following sections describe how to use Outlook Express to participate in newsgroups.

Subscribing to a newsgroup

The benefit of subscribing is that the newsgroup is included in your 'folders' list for easy access. You can subscribe to a newsgroup in several ways. When you add a news server, Outlook Express prompts you to subscribe to newsgroups on that server. Click a news server name in your 'folders' list, and then click the 'newsgroups' button. Select the newsgroup that you want to subscribe to, and then click the 'subscribe' button. You can also unsubscribe here. When you double-click a name in the 'newsgroup' list, a subscription is automatically generated. When you view a newsgroup without subscribing to it, its name appears in your 'folders' list. Right-click the name and then click 'subscribe'.

To view a newsgroup to which you subscribe, click it in the 'folders' list. To cancel your subscription to a newsgroup, click the 'newsgroups' button, click the 'subscribed' tab, select the group you want, and then click the 'unsubscribe' button. You can also right click the newsgroup in your 'folders' list and then click 'unsubscribe'.

How to post messages to a newsgroup

There are several ways that you can post messages, depending on whether you are posting a new message or replying to one and how widely you want it distributed. You can also format messages, and add your signature, business card, or links to files.

In the 'folders' list select the newsgroup to which you want to post a message. On the toolbar, click the 'new post' button. To send your message to multiple newsgroups on the same news server, click the icon next to 'newsgroups' in the 'new message' dialogue box. In the 'pick news groups' dialogue box, click one or more newsgroups from the list (hold down the CTRL key to select multiple newsgroups) and then click 'add'. You can choose from all newsgroups, or only those you subscribe to, by clicking the 'show only subscribed newsgroups' button. Type the subject of your message and, when completed, click the 'send' button.

You can send a message to more than one newsgroup at a time only if all the newsgroups are on the same news server. To post a message to newsgroups on other news servers, create a separate message for each news server.

You can cancel a message you have posted by selecting the message, clicking the 'message' menu and then selecting 'cancel message'. Cancelling a message does not remove it from a newsgroup user's computer if the user downloaded the message before it was cancelled. You can cancel only messages you have posted; you cannot cancel another person's message.

To reply to a newsgroup message

In the message list, click on the message to which you want to reply. To reply to the author of the message by e-mail, click the 'reply' button on the toolbar. To reply to the whole newsgroup, click the 'reply group' button on the toolbar.

If you want your reply to go to additional newsgroups on the same news server, click the icon next to 'newsgroups' in the 'reply' dialogue box. In the 'pick newsgroups' dialogue box, select a newsgroup from the list, and then click 'add'. You can choose from all newsgroups or only those you subscribe to by clicking the 'show only subscribed newsgroups' button. Type your message and then click 'send'. You can send your reply to more than one newsgroup at a time only if all the newsgroups are on the same news server.

To view information about a newsgroup message, such as when it was sent, select the message, click 'file'/'properties'. A dialogue box will be displayed containing information about the message.

To send large messages

Many mail and news servers limit the size of the messages you can receive and send. Usually this limit is one megabyte (1 MB) per message, including all attached files. With Outlook Express, however, you can send large messages or files to mail and news servers that have size limits by breaking the messages into smaller ones. When the group of messages is received, the e-mail program recombines them into one message.

1. Click 'tools'/'accounts'.
2. On either the mail or news tab, click 'properties'.
3. On the 'advanced' tab, select the 'break apart' messages larger than 'x' KB check box and then enter the maximum file size the server will allow.

To find messages in a newsgroup

While in a newsgroup, click the 'edit' menu, point to 'find', and then select 'message in this folder'. In the 'look for text' box, type the word(s) you want to search for and then click 'find next'. If your search returns too many results or does not give you what you want, click the 'advanced find' button and type in as much information as possible to refine your search.

You can also find messages by sorting the columns (clicking the 'subject', 'from', or 'sent' heads and so on). Click the column heading to reorder the messages in that column. For example, when you click the 'from' column, messages are sorted alphabetically by the sender's name.

To group together messages and their replies

When many people participate in e-mail and newsgroup conversations, the replies to a given message can be hard to track. You can set up Outlook Express so that message replies are grouped under the original message. You can then choose to view only the original message, or the message and all its replies.

When you are in either your 'inbox' or a newsgroup, click the 'view' menu, then 'current view' and select 'group messages by conversation'. To display expanded conversations for all messages, click the 'tools' menu, click 'options', click the 'read' tab, and then select the 'automatically expand grouped messages' check box.

To display the original message and all replies to it, click the plus sign to the left of the original message. To display only the original message, click the minus sign next to the message. Conversations are grouped according to the title of the original message. For example, if the message that starts a conversation is titled 'qualitative methodologies' all replies to that message will be titled 'qualitative methodologies'.

To set up newsgroups for offline news reading

You can set up Outlook Express to make messages or headers in the newsgroups to which you subscribe available offline by synchronizing. This enables you to read them at your leisure when you are off-line. From the 'folders' list, select a news server. In the main window, select one or more newsgroups you subscribe to whose messages you want to read 'off-line'. Click the 'settings' button and then click a selection, marking what you want transferred from the server to your computer during synchronization. The options will be something like: 'all messages; new messages only' (new to the server since you last synchronized); 'headers only' (subject, author, date, and size of message). Make sure that the newsgroups you do not want to download are not checked (don't synchronize). Whenever you want to transfer the messages or headers to your computer from the server, click the 'sync account' button.

To download individual messages

You can specify certain messages within a newsgroup for download the next time you connect by selecting the headers you want while offline. While offline, select the previously downloaded message headers required. In the 'tools' menu, select 'mark for offline', and then click 'download message later'. Repeat for each newsgroup whose messages you want to read later. When you go online, on the 'tools' menu, click 'synchronize all', and then go 'offline' after your messages are downloaded.

You can display only the messages that you selected for 'offline' reading. After you download the messages for 'offline' reading and disconnect (go off-line), click the 'view' menu and select 'current view'/'show downloaded messages'. Be aware that there are a lot of groups that send pornographic images to your computer. The title of such a newsgroup gives a strong indication of its content. Downloading these images is likely to be breaking the law. If in doubt do not subscribe to the newsgroup.

Spam

Spam is the term given to unwanted e-mail messages. These can be unsolicited advertising or worse, such as pornographic e-mail attachments. Remember, some people also send mail containing viruses so it is necessary both to check all mail and downloads for viruses and to set up your system to block or filter unwanted mail. Do not reply to unwanted mail as it just confirms to the sender that there is someone reading the inbox and encourages them to send more mail.

You can control the-mail and news messages you get in Outlook Express in several ways. You can block certain people from sending you mail, you can hide conversations that don't interest you, and you can guard against being sent damaging code in mail by setting security levels.

To block messages, all that you have to do is select the e-mail message in the Outlook Express window, click on 'message'/'block sender' and the address will be added automatically to a list of blocked senders. To view that list click on the menu 'tools'/'message rules'/'block senders list'. A small dialogue tab box will appear and you can add other e-mail addresses to the list by clicking on the 'add' button and typing the address in the blank field displayed. You then choose whether to block mail, news, or mail and news messages. Click the OK button to complete the action.

Netiquette (e-mail etiquette)

There are informal conventions about the contents of an e-mail. These conventions are basically courtesy measures. To aid the art of e-mail communications, users developed a system of characters using different combinations of keyboard characters that represent human emotions. These characters are called smileys, or emoticons. A smiley is read by leaning your head toward your left shoulder and looking at the characters sideways, reading from left to right. Some examples are:

A happy face :-)
A sad face :-(
Wears glasses 8-)
Wears braces :-#
Smokes a pipe :-?
Has a moustache :-{
Winking/sarcastic ;-)
Undecided :-\
Oops :-o

It is fun to add them to messages. Be aware that SHOUTING is represented by typing in capital letters. Emphasis is added to a word by adding underscore before and after words, for example '_emphasis_'.

You might also see abbreviations used in e-mail. Some are listed below:

BTW – by the way
c-ya – see you later
FAQ – frequently asked questions
FWIW – for what it's worth
IMHO – in my humble opinion
LOL – laughing out loud
OTOH – on the other hand
TIA – thanks in advance

Practice

Log on to the two following discussion list sites: http://www.liszt.com and http://www.jiscmail.ac.uk. Select a group from each and subscribe to them. If you are unsure about what to do there should be additional instructions available via a link on the home page of the sites.

An e-mail will be sent to you at the address that you specify when you subscribed. A typical introductory message is as in the following example:

Wed, 13 Jan 1999 06:18:39

Your subscription to the OJNI-L list (Online Journal of Nursing Informatics) has been accepted.

Please save this message for future reference, especially if this is the first time you subscribe to an electronic mailing list. If you ever need to leave the list, you will find the necessary instructions below. Perhaps more importantly, saving a copy of this message (and of all future subscription notices from other mailing lists) in a special mail folder will give you instant access to the list of mailing lists that you are subscribed to. This may prove very useful the next time you go on vacation and need to leave the lists temporarily so as not to fill up your mailbox while you are away! You should also save the 'welcome messages' from the list owners that you will occasionally receive after subscribing to a new list.

To send a message to all the people currently subscribed to the list, just send mail to OJNI-L@LISTS.PSU.EDU. This is called 'sending mail to the list', because you send mail to a single address and LISTSERV makes copies for all the people who have subscribed. This address (OJNI-L@LISTS.PSU.EDU) is also called the 'list address'. You must never try to send any command to that address, as it would be distributed to all the people who have subscribed. All commands must be sent to the 'LISTSERV address', LISTSERV@LISTS.PSU.EDU. It is very important to understand the difference between the two, but fortunately it is not complicated. The LISTSERV address is like a FAX number that connects you to a machine, whereas the list address is like a normal voice line connecting you to a person. If you make a mistake and dial the FAX number when you wanted to talk to someone on the phone, you will quickly realize that you used the wrong number and call again. No harm will have been done. If on the other hand you accidentally make your FAX call someone's voice line, the person receiving the call will be inconvenienced, especially if your FAX then re-dials every 5 minutes. The fact that most people will eventually connect the FAX machine to the voice line to allow the FAX to go through and make the calls stop does not mean that you should continue to send FAXes to the voice number. People would just get mad at you. It works pretty much the same way with mailing lists, with the difference that you are calling hundreds or thousands of people at the same time, and consequently you can expect a lot of people to get upset if you consistently send commands to the list address.

You may leave the list at any time by sending a 'SIGNOFF OJNI-L' command to LISTSERV@LISTS.PSU.EDU. You can also tell LISTSERV how you want it to confirm the receipt of messages you send to the list. If you do not trust the system, send a 'SET OJNI-L REPRO' command and LISTSERV will send you a copy of your own messages, so that you can see that the message was distributed and did not get damaged on the way. After a while you may find that this is getting annoying, especially if your mail program does not tell you that the message is from you when it informs you that new mail has arrived from OJNI-L. If you send a 'SET OJNI-L ACK NOREPRO' command, LISTSERV will mail you a short acknowledgement instead, which will look different in your mailbox directory. With most mail programs you will know

(contd)

immediately that this is an acknowledgement you can read later. Finally, you can turn off acknowledgements completely with 'SET OJNI-L NOACK NOREPRO'.

Following instructions from the list owner, your subscription options have been set to 'REPRO MIME' rather than the usual LISTSERV defaults. For more information about subscription options, send a 'QUERY OJNI-L' command to LISTSERV@LISTS.PSU.EDU.

This list is available in digest form. If you wish to receive the digested version of the postings, just issue a SET OJNI-L DIGEST command. Please note that it is presently possible for other people to determine that you are signed up to the list through the use of the 'REVIEW' command, which returns the e-mail address and name of all the subscribers. If you do not want your name to be visible, just issue a 'SET OJNI-L CONCEAL' command. More information on LIST-SERV commands can be found in the LISTSERV reference card, which you can retrieve by sending an 'INFO REFCARD' command to LISTSERV@LISTS.PSU.EDU.

Once e-mails start to arrive in your inbox spend some time 'lurking' to get a feel for the character of the list. Read previous threads too and, once you feel ready to contribute, post a message.

Chapter 8
Making sense of electronic information

Now that you have developed your information searching skills, this final chapter suggests some ways to make sense of the information that you find on the Internet. The analysis of research papers is a subject in its own right but there still remains a critical approach to Web-based information that helps you to evaluate its worth. The following is synthesized from a number of articles that deal with this topic. Their URLs are provided so that you can read the full text online.

A guide to critiquing Web-based information

You need to evaluate the following in order to assess information that you find on the WWW:

Authorship

- Who is the author?
- What are his or her credentials?
- When was the article first published?
- When was it posted on the web?
- Has it been reviewed since first publication?
- Is this a revision?
- Is the author identified with a particular discipline?
- Does the author reveal any particular purpose for writing this material?

Publication

- What is the title of the journal in which the material is published?
- Is the site sponsor identifiable?
- Who is the intended audience?
- Is this a peer-reviewed piece of work?
- Is it scholarly or non-scholarly?
- Can the work be retrieved from a paper-based source too or is it only in electronic format?
- How is the information presented?
- Does it support statements made or does it major on opinion?
- Is the information accurate?
- What are the sources cited to support the content of the material?
- Is there attention to style, grammar and spelling?

Site design

- Is the site easy to navigate?
- Does the site have any indication of a periodic review to maintain the quality of presentation and content?
- Does it have an auto-notification facility regarding updates?
- Are the links to pages within the site or to outside of the site?
- Are these links periodically checked to ensure that they work?
- Is there any indication of review of the rationale for selecting links connected to this site?

If you are viewing a research paper you will need to consider not only who the authors are and what discipline they represent but also who has sponsored the research. Why they are writing and who is their intended audience? The kind of journal in which the material is found will give a good indication of this and the guidelines for authors will set out the intended readership of the journal. You should also consider:

- the research focus
- the research question or hypothesis
- why this particular question is being asked at this time
- the literature cited to explain the context
- the selection of appropriate methodology and methods of data collection

- issues of access, ethics and sampling
- the duration of data collection and the method of analysis of data
- the presentation of results and findings
- whether the discussion draws valid conclusions from the data
- whether or not the findings are discussed in the light of the context provided
- whether the research process is replicable (can it be repeated?) and, if replicated, whether the same conclusions would be likely to be drawn
- whether there is sufficient information provided to replicate the study.

You might also look at a BMJ article about reading a paper at http://www.bmj.com/collections/read.shtml.

The key issue with any information that you retrieve is to make a judgement about its value to your enquiry. Sometimes it will be sufficient to view abstracts of articles and decide whether they are useful or not useful. It is essential to develop the skill of identifying material that matches your enquiry and, if it is irrelevant, to discard it in favour of something that is relevant. The danger of not doing so is that you might waste a lot of valuable time surfing around the Internet, without progressing your enquiry very much.

Articles exploring critical appraisal of Web-based information

Several articles on the Internet discuss the critical appraisal of Web-based information:

- Jackson T, Cohen L. Evaluating Internet Resources: http://www.albany.edu/library/internet/evaluate.html
- McGonigle D. How to Evaluate Web Sites: http://cac.psu.edu/~dxm12/siteval.html
- Grassian E. Thinking Critically about World Wide Web Resources: http://www.library.ucla.edu/libraries/college/instruct/web/critical.htm
- Harris R. Evaluating Internet Research Sources: http://www.vanguard.edu/rharris/evalu8it.htm

Web addresses (URLs) do alter and some material is removed from servers. If these links no longer exist then find a plain text metasearch engine such as Ask Jeeves (http://www.ask.co.uk) and search for 'critical review of Internet resources'.

Conclusion

There remains much that could be said about the introduction of IT into the workplace, the advent of healthcare record systems such as the electronic health record and the provision of real time information. This book represents a start, an initial experience in this vast and technological field. However, it should equip you with sufficient 'know-how' to enable you to use the available technology effectively.

The following selected Web sites will help to support your professional practice. Many other helpful sites are available on the Internet and you will no doubt develop a personal directory of sites around your own area of interest.

- UK government web site: http://www.open.gov.uk
- World Health Organization: http://who.org
- Higher Education Statistics Agency: http://hesa.ac.uk/
- The Academic Directory: http://acdc.hensa.ac.uk/index.shtml
- NHS IM & T electronic library links page: http://www.standards.nhsia.nhs.uk/library/links.htm
- NHS Centre for Reviews and Dissemination: http://www.york.ac.uk/inst/crd/
- NHS Executive Publications: http://www.doh.gov.uk/nhspub.htm
- NICE: http://www.nice.org.uk
- Evidence-based Medicine Journals: http://www.ebmny.org/journal.html
- Introduction to Evidence-based Medicine: http://www.hsl.unc.edu/EBM/welcome.htm
- Evidence-based Medicine Resource Centre: http://www.ebmny.org/
- POEMS: http://www.infopoems.com/
- Bandolier homepage: http://www.ebando.com/
- US National Library of Medicine: http://www.nlm.nih.gov/
- Virtual Library Medicine and Health:

http://www.vlib.org/Medicine.html
- Medline: http://www.nlm.nih.gov/medlineplus/databases.html
- Web of Science: http://wos.mimas.ac.uk/
- Social Science Information Gateway:
  SOSIG.http://www.sosig.ac.uk/
- Sociological Research Online:
  http://www.socresonline.org.uk/info/style.html
- Findarticles.com: http://www.findarticles.com
- The Data Protection Act:
  http://www.hmso.gov.uk/acts/acts1998/19980029.htm

Glossary

Antivirus software a program that detects and will clean viruses from a PC. There are various antivirus software programs on the market such as Norton, VET and Dr. Solomon.

Backup to backup data is to make a copy onto disk or tape of whatever is on the computer's hard drive. A single file can be backed up or the whole hard drive.

Bits and bytes a bit is the smallest unit of information that computers can handle. A group of eight bits is called a byte and this is the unit used for describing the memory capacity of the computers hard disk.. e.g. 850 megabytes is 850 million bytes.

Boot up the process of starting up a computer and waiting for it to work through various programs until it is ready for use is called booting up. The instructions to boot up are stored on a boot disk you should make a recovery boot disk copy in case you have problems booting up your system. The boot disk is normally the PCs hard disk.

Browser a browser is a program used to view information on the internet. Current examples are Microsoft® Internet Explorer and Netscape Navigator.

Bug a name for a fault or some other defect in a computer system.

Cache a section of memory devoted to speeding up the operation of the computer. Some processor chips have a cache incorporated, others have the cache separate, on the motherboard.

CD Rom compact disk read only memory. A disc containing information which can be read, but not altered in the way a floppy disk can be. *See* CD Rom re-write.

CPU central processing unit. This is the computer's processor and is akin the the brain of the computer. The world's largest maufacturer of processors is Intel who make the Pentium processor.

DOS disk operating system. This was a system which enabled the PC to function. To use it required knowledge of the right commands to type in. Examples were IBM OS2 and Microsoft DOS 6. Applications were then loaded to 'sit' on the operating system such as Microsoft works. This has been superceded by modern operating systems such as Windows.

Driver a program which the computer needs to tell it how a particular application works. A printer for example will come with a driver to load into the PC so that the computer system can know how to link up to that particular model.

Electronic mail / e-mail mail sent from one computer to another and which can either be read on screen or printed out.

Expansion slots a PCs motherboard has slots built into it which allow other pieces of hardware to be added such as plug-in cards. There are different designs of slot depending upon the age of the motherboard and changing industry standards. Examples are PCI and ISA and VESA.

Floppy disk a floppy disk is a removable disk used for storage of information. It is a disc of magnetic material and is now a standard 3.5" size and usually comes with a storage capacity of 1.44 megabytes [MB]. They need to be formatted before use or can be purchased pre-formatted. It looks like a plastic square with a thin metal slide covering an opening on one side.

File a small amount of specific information such as a letter that will be kept in a folder.

Folder the vast amount of information stored on hard disks is usually stored in smaller subdivisions of information called folders. They contain related items which make it easier to locate information.

Font a font is the style of lettering used in typing text. Examples are Times New Roman and Arial.

Format before a floppy or hard disk can be used to store information it has to be electronically prepared or formatted. If a floppy disk is not formatted there will be a program on your computer which will allow you to do this. Be careful of reformatting your hard disk as this will clear all the information on it. Make sure that you have a backup, and do not reformat your hard disk if you are not sure what you are doing.

Gb gigabyte, which is a thousand million bytes.

Graphics card a plug-in card inside the PC which generates the picture you see on the screen. The larger the memory size of the graphics card the greater the handling of images and colours. To handle modern games in 3 dimensions you will need at least a 4MB card, otherwise the pictures will appear to jump as opposed to smooth 3 Dimensional scrolling.

Hard drive the metal disc which is inside the computer and looks like a rectangular metal box on which PC information and programs are stored. It may help to think of it as a filing cabinet in which many files are stored. Some portable computers have removable hard drives.

Icon a picture on the computer screen that acts as a symbol for folders and other objects.

IDE a common type of hard disk.

Internet a worldwide network of computers which can be accessed via telephone or satellite links. It is also called the world wide web (www).

ISA a type of expansion slot on a motherboard.

Kb kilobyte - a thousand bytes.

Mb megabyte - a million bytes.

Memory memory is used to temporarily store information such as programs and data whilst the computer is in use.

MHz megahertz. The term used to describe the speed at which a computer processor operates. The higher the speed the better. A few years ago 33MHz was fast, now we are looking at 450MHz and beyond.

Modem an internal or external piece of hardware allowing the computer to send digital information down telephone lines. If you are reading this online then you will be using a modem somewhere in your computer system.

Motherboard the main circuit board of the computer onto which the CPU, plug-in cards, drives and memory are fitted.

Parallel port a socket in the back of a PC for connecting external equipment such as a printer.

PC card a credit sized card which can be plugged into a slot on a notebook computer. Modems, memory and hard disks can all be in the form of PC cards.

PCI a type of expansion slot on a motherboard.

Pentium a processor used in computers. There are different versions such as Intel, MMX and Celeron.

Peripheral a piece of equipment which is connected to the computer, such as a mouse.

Pixel a computer screen image is made up of thousands of dots. Each one is a pixel. The more pixels per inch the higher the resolution of the image.

Plug and play Window's type systems have a feature where newly added equipment is automatically recognised by the computer and adjustments made.

Program a piece of software which give instructions to the PC to do a particular set of tasks.

RAM Random Access Memory, a type of memory used by the computer as workspace whilst it is operating. VRAM is video memory dedicated to producing the screen image.

Resolution the term given to the number of pixels used to produce an image on the screen and is expressed as dots horizontally and vertically. An example is SVGA 800x600 pixels.

ROM read only memory filled with key information required by the computer that cannot be altered.

Scanner a piece of equipment which converts paper documents into electronic pictures understood by the PC. Beware of copywrite restrictions on the electronic storage of data. Scanners are either flatbed, hand held or incorporated in a printer.

SCSI small computer systems interface. An alternative to the IDE for connecting hard drives and peripherals.

Serial port a socket on the back of the PC used to connect external equipment such as a mouse.

SIMM single in line memory module. A group of memory chips mounted on a plug in motherboard.

SVGA *See* resolution.

Taskbar a feature of Window's screens. It usually has a 'start' button in the bottom left hand corner which, when clicked on, pops up a menu of options.

TFT thin film transistor. A type of flat screen used on notebooks to provide high quality pictures.

Virus the term given to a range of programs which can infect your computer and alter or totally stop its operation. They are introduced via loading software or from the internet. It is essential to have up to date anti-virus software and to keep backups of data.

Windows an operating system which uses a graphical approach combining keyboard and mouse controls. Programs can be operated by pointing the mouse at them on the screen (e.g. an icon) and clicking on them.

WYSIWYG what you see is what you get. The picture on the screen is what you get when printing it.

Index